MW00813901

ADVANCE PRAISE

"*Dr. Bhanote's in-depth knowledge of nutrition and medicine—including the surprising connections between mind and body—will empower you to overcome whatever challenges have kept you from reaching your health goals. Her holistic approach is exciting, powerful, and revolutionary.*"

NEAL D. BARNARD, MD, President of the Physicians Committee for Responsible Medicine and author of *Your Body in Balance: The New Science of Food, Hormones, and Health*

"*In The Anatomy of Wellbeing, Dr. Monisha Bhanote leads readers into better health and vibrancy and increased longevity. Through educating about health from the cellular level to the mind-body-spirit connection, she presents health information in an inspiring and motivational way. Enjoy the multidimensional approach. There is something for everyone in this book.*"

ANN MARIE CHIASSON, MD, associate professor at the Andrew Weil Center for Integrative Medicine and author of *Energy Healing: The Essentials of Self-Care*

"The Anatomy of Wellbeing *is the book we've all been needing. Dr. Bhanote has taken us on a journey through the inner workings of the human body and how our daily lifestyle practices can be utilized to enhance our optimal state of being.*"

TIFFANY CRUIKSHANK, L.AC, Founder of Yoga Medicine
and author of *Optimal Health for a Vibrant Life*

"*Quite simply,* The Anatomy of Wellbeing *is an organizing framework to put your mind, body, and entire lifestyle together into one view for your greater experience of health and wellness. Dr. Bhanote has made the complex workings of the human body both practical and relatable so you can start taking action to feel your best today.*"

STEVEN GURGEVICH, PHD, author of *The Self-Hypnosis Diet*

"*Finally, an intelligent guidebook that speaks to how the body works and how I can continue to break the glass ceiling not only in business but also with my own health. Dr. Bhanote's* The Anatomy of Wellbeing *has made me reevaluate what I can do to improve my own wellbeing and take a proactive role.*"

HEATHER MONAHAN, bestselling author of *Overcome Your Villains*

"*Dr. Monisha Bhanote is uniquely qualified to dispense a holistic approach to whole-body healing with intentional practices that will support your physical and mental wellbeing.*"

LISE ALSCHULER, ND, co-author of
The Definitive Guide to Thriving After Cancer

"*In* The Anatomy of Wellbeing, *Dr. Bhanote combines her years of experience in both conventional medicine and integrative health to present a comprehensive exploration of the human body. She skillfully weaves together daily rituals for wellness, inviting readers on a priceless journey toward uncovering their inner vibrance and whole health.*"

RASHMI BISMARK, MD, MPH, author of *Finding Om*

"*Dr. Bhanote has done an impressive job of highlighting the importance of a functional body to both prevent disease and enhance longevity.* The Anatomy of Wellbeing *will become your go-to guide for a whole-body approach to health and happiness.*"

SHONA ELLIOTT, author of *Creating Value as a Senior Leader*

"The Anatomy of Wellbeing *is for anyone who really needs a full-body approach to taking action on their health and happiness. My colleague Dr. Monisha Bhanote has taken years of her medical expertise to lay out a contemporary plan that anyone can use to feel empowered to start moving their health in the right direction.*"

RAJ DASGUPTA, MD, author of
Medicine Morning Report: Beyond the Pearls

"*This book delivers the most practical and straightforward health and wellness information I have ever read.*"

DR. SAM BERNE, Founder of Holistic Eye Care

"The Anatomy of Wellbeing: Intentional Practices to Embrace Your Body's Unique Design and Revitalize Your Health *by Dr. Monisha Bhanote is more than just a clinician's view of the state of healthcare and medicine. It's a journey with guidance along the way to empower each of us, as we are each responsible for our own health and wellness. She provides practical tools and practices for everyday life to take small, intentional, incremental changes toward improved health and wellbeing. This book is not just a 'read and you're done' publication; it's an ongoing reference for our own journeys in health and happiness.*"

DENNIS AND KATHY LANG, authors of *Everything Matters*

"*In this book, Dr. Monisha Bhanote empowers people by educating them about how to take care of their health on a cellular level. She provides a step-by-step, sustainable roadmap for anyone wishing to achieve their optimal health. She shows you how to follow habits that are nourishing to every cell of your body and provides science-backed reasons! If you are ready to optimize your health, this is the book for you!*"

BOJANA JANKOVIC WEATHERLY, MD, FACP, MSc, IFMCP, FORBES HEALTH MEDICAL ADVISORY BOARD MEMBER

THE
ANATOMY
OF
WELLBEING

THE
ANATOMY
OF
WELLBEING

Intentional Practices
to Embrace Your Body's Unique Design
and Revitalize Your Health

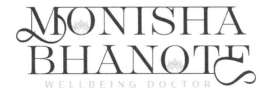

MONISHA
BHANOTE
WELLBEING DOCTOR

The content in this book represents the research and ideas of its author and is intended to supplement, not replace, the advice of qualified health professionals. Prior to starting any diet or other medical regimen, consult your health care provider. This book's author and publisher expressly disclaim all liability, loss, or risk, whether direct or indirect, resulting from the use and application of its contents.

In the absence of permission, scanning, uploading, and disseminating this book constitutes theft of the author's intellectual property. For permission to use material from the book (other than for review purposes), please contact TAOW@drbhanote.com. Thank you for supporting the rights of the author.

Images are courtesy of the author.

LIONCREST
PUBLISHING

THE ANATOMY OF WELLBEING
Intentional Practices to Embrace Your Body's Unique Design and Revitalize Your Health

ISBN 978-1-5445-3455-8 *Hardcover*

978-1-5445-3456-5 *Paperback*

978-1-5445-3457-2 *Ebook*

CONTENTS

YOUR WELLBEING

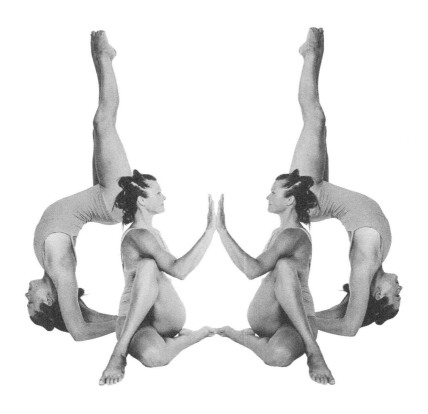

JOURNEY BEGINS HERE

*This book is dedicated to all those
interested in naturally biohacking their consciousness.*

*Let this book inspire you to live with intention,
embrace a sustainable lifestyle,
and transform your wellbeing.*

INTRODUCTION

*"Never underestimate the power you have to take your
life in a new direction."*

~ GERMANY KENT, AUTHOR AND JOURNALIST

EVERY PATIENT WHO COMES TO MY OFFICE HAS A STORY—ONE
as unique as their own anatomy, individual habits, and lifestyles.

There's the successful career woman who can't find time to work
out or cook her meals, so she opts for fast meals over healthy ones.
She knows that her health is on a slow decline as her anxiety climbs
and her energy decreases.

There's the forty-year-old bachelor trying to come to grips with the
fact that he can't eat or party the way he did in his twenties, who
can't understand why his cholesterol is so high, even though he
does CrossFit five days a week.

There's the young college student who wonders why his protein
shakes aren't helping him put on muscle, who constantly struggles
to focus and remember material for his tests.

1

Then there's the cancer survivor who wants to purge her life of every potential cancer-causing agent—and hopefully, find ways to improve her quality of life while doing it.

Every person's story is different, but at the end of the day, we all want the same thing: to feel well, *be* well, and perform at our best. We recognize that some variable in our lifestyle might be hindering us from achieving those goals, but we don't know what. Many of us are tired of the Band-Aid solutions offered through quick appointments and even quicker prescriptions. Instead, we want to get to the bottom of what's going on in our bodies.

I speak to people like this—perhaps people like *you*—every day. They come to me with their questions, and slowly, we begin putting the pieces together. We look at their lifestyle, their diet, their bloodwork, and their presenting symptoms. There is no "one size fits all" approach. I teach my patients how their bodies work, what damages their cells, and what their bodies need to thrive. After decades of practicing medicine, this information feels familiar to me, but I'm always surprised to see it isn't common knowledge to everyone. I see lightbulbs go off for my patients when they learn some new, interesting fact about their bodies. "What?!" they'll ask me incredulously. "Why didn't I learn that in school? Everyone needs to know this!"

"I know!" I'll agree with them. "They *do*. Everyone should know this!"

#CellCare: A holistic approach to wellbeing is having your body and mind functioning optimally.

OUR COLLECTIVE "DIS-EASE"

It's no secret: we are unwell. The word *disease* spells this out: *dis* means a lack of, and *ease* refers to ease or health. Disease previously described lacking comfort. Now, of course, it has come to mean a state of illness and deviation from our optimal state. In either case, we are good descriptions of the word *disease*. In America, we're more anxious than ever, we have more chronic health issues than ever, and more than 40 percent of Americans are clinically obese.[1] One in four millennials has a chronic disease, such as high cholesterol, high blood pressure, and diabetes.[2] We are struggling to sleep, and we're too overloaded to focus. Most of us are in a bad mood much of the time: we're irritable, short-tempered, and depressed, and the cells in our body are *angry* and asking us to take care of them.

True, we're *living* longer than ever—but the extension of our lifespan made possible by modern medicine doesn't mean we're healthy and happy. Unfortunately, many people accept it as a given that they'll probably need a plethora of medications to get through the day by the time they are older.

However, others are pushing back. They know their lifestyle is a significant factor in their wellbeing, and they're ready to implement practices—they just don't know what to do.

Worldwide, the wellness industry has a value of $4.5 *trillion*.[3] On the one hand, that's a good indication that many people in the world are ready to invest in their wellbeing. On the other hand, it means there are vast amounts of misinformation out there. There are plenty of ineffective health products dressed up with good advertising, not to mention many so-called "experts" giving people recommendations that are not effective or grounded in science. It can be challenging to determine what information is legitimate.

Another challenge comes from a failure to connect the dots. Most people have vague ideas that they should eat better, exercise more, or prioritize their mental health. Still, they struggle to put in the time and effort—mainly because it's hard to clearly *see* the impact of their lifestyle choices on their bodies. People are confused about what options will conclusively affect their health. For example, a person might have watched their parent battle with dementia or cope with diabetes, but they can't identify all the factors leading to their parent's struggle. So why would they change anything in their own lives until they're in the same position? There's no clear line connecting the dots between lifestyle factors and chronic disease diagnosis. That can make it hard for people to prioritize healthy lifestyle changes.

Unfortunately, the solutions offered by conventional care often fall short. Patients seek me out as an integrative and functional medicine physician because they have grown impatient with the siloed approach of medicine. They have one doctor for this problem, another doctor for that problem, and a host of prescriptions that might be working against each other. In addition, our current healthcare system tends to focus on symptom management, not preventative care. Anyone looking to address a complicated or confusing health issue—or anyone looking to avoid the need for prescriptions in the first place—can find this incredibly frustrating.

My philosophy is that medicine should aim to do more than alleviate symptoms and prevent death; it should also discover the underlying cause of disease and increase *healthspan*. As a result, we should treat the entire body, acknowledging the link between mind, body, and spirit. The phrase "integrative and functional medicine" hints that it aims to help a person function optimally and integrate well-being in all areas of life. The patient should be an active participant in their care, and their personalized care should promote optimal health, reverse disease, and improve quality of life. A whole-body approach requires attention to more than just physical symptoms; it recognizes that health also involves your mental wellness, nutrition, physical movement, and so on.

Yet even when we have the correct information with solutions, it can still be challenging to make necessary changes to your lifestyle. It's not unusual for people to throw themselves into a new healthy lifestyle for a few weeks, only to find they can't sustain it. The necessary changes just seem too difficult. They return to their old habits with a new sense of futility.

I hear about it. I see it—I've even lived it. But the story doesn't end there.

THE JOURNEY TOWARD WELLBEING

Living a life of wellbeing is not about quick fixes. It's a journey that starts at birth and lasts until our last breath. So, our journey toward health, happiness, and wellbeing will be a lifelong practice. And that's okay!

When taking the long view regarding your wellbeing, making small changes actually becomes more manageable. During your journey, you will not feel as threatened by the setbacks and challenges you might experience in your health; you will understand that each hurdle is simply a new turn. It's okay for your body to change over time—it might just need unique aspects of TLC from you to ensure it continues to thrive.

The secret to doing this is "#CellCare." Your body is composed of some 37.2 trillion cells, each with their own structure and function. Your health will depend on how you take care of these cells. Throughout this book, I will discuss ways you can help your cells remain healthy and aligned so that they can function optimally. First, we'll discuss the ingredients your body needs to operate smoothly so that your cells stay happy and don't become *angry* at you. Then, we'll pursue greater alignment—covering the mind, body, and spirit—so that your cells can travel the path of least resistance toward health. When your cells can function at their best, *you* can function at your best. In that way, #CellCare is the most natural form of self-care.

> **#CellCare:** Self-healing requires cellular healing.

I remember when I first bought a brand-new car. I loved how shiny and new everything felt. But over time, my car needed maintenance. For its engine to work well, the oil needed to be regularly changed; the tires needed rotation; it needed to be washed; and sometimes, the car needed an extensive repair. Your body requires maintenance too. You can get a new vehicle, but you can't exactly trade in your body! The earlier you understand that you need to practice #CellCare for your body and mind proactively, the more likely you will ensure wellbeing in your future years.

It's also crucial to understand that when it comes to your body, everything is connected. Your mind connects to your gut, which connects to your immune system, which connects to the blood that flows to all your organs. I could go on and on about this, and in fact, I will, throughout the rest of this book with many science-based recommendations. If you want to optimize your health and wellbeing, you will want to take a whole-body approach. You don't just need a bottle of pills. You need a comprehensive lifestyle practice. Moreover, you need one that feels *easy* and is *sustainable.*

Sometimes we think that spurts of activity will influence our health—we go to the gym once and suddenly expect that to make a change in our lives. That gym session might help you feel good in the short term, but it's not likely to help you achieve your long-term goals. You eat a big salad for the week, and you feel you have given your body what it needs. In reality, health and wellness will be determined by whatever you do *most of the time*—not *some* of the time. The small, intentional changes I recommend will enable you to build a consistent and sustainable lifestyle oriented toward wellbeing.

> **#CellCare:** Living an intentional, sustainable lifestyle that is tailored to your personal goals is the first step on the journey to wellbeing.

Maybe that still sounds too hard. If you prefer to maintain your current lifestyle, regardless of what it's doing to your body, and coast on whatever pharmaceuticals your doctor prescribes when your body declines, then I give you permission to put this book down. It's not for you at this time.

This book is for people with a genuine curiosity about how their bodies work, people who hear recommendations like, "Eat more vegetables," and automatically ask *why*? It's for people who know in the back of their mind that they could be living better—and *want* to be living better—they just need to know where to start.

If that sounds like you, then be encouraged. Every single chapter in this book will put you ahead of where you were the day before.

THE PATH TO REVITALIZATION

Step by step, this book will guide you through the different facets of your lifestyle that directly affect your wellbeing. With simple, straightforward explanations, you will walk through the anatomy at play behind each element of your lifestyle. For instance, you'll learn precisely how sleep impacts your mental and physical health and is integral to repairing your cells. You will learn to optimize digestion so your body makes the hormones and neurotransmitters it needs to function at its best. Each chapter will conclude with a series of intentional practices—what I call rituals—that can help you make small changes in a way that embraces your body's unique design.

Your path to revitalization will become increasingly clear as you progress through your journey to wellbeing and become better acquainted with your whole body. Here is where your journey begins:

◆ **Power of rituals:** Incorporating the science of neuroplasticity, you will learn how to transform your mind and body through small, sustainable, intentional changes. These concepts will inform your understanding of each subsequent chapter. By following my strategies, you will be able to implement these practices effectively and purposefully.

◆ **Transforming your mindset:** Your mindset governs what happens in your body—and how your mind and body respond to experiences. You will gain insight into the anatomy of your stress response and tools to embrace a growth mindset. As a result, the changes outlined in the following chapters will be easier to implement.

◆ **Your body's ecosystem:** Your health and wellbeing are greatly influenced by the health and function of your cells. By knowing how your body functions and the nutrients it requires for optimal health, you can make informed decisions about your health. Upon learning how everything within your body is connected, it will become apparent why you want to take good care of your cells.

◆ **Culinary nourishment:** What you eat affects your mood, cognition, and wellbeing. Food can be medicine—yet many people are unaware of which foods provide their bodies with the nutrients they need to thrive. You will learn about nutritional science and culinary medicine to better understand your digestion, uncomplicate nutrition, and discover which nutrients you should consume regularly.

- **Art of movement:** There is no doubt that your body is designed to move—and the movements you make can have incredibly positive effects. You will learn about the different types of movements most beneficial for your body and the amazing results they can have on your cellular health.

- **Restorative recovery:** Sleep is one of the greatest gifts you can give to your body, as it impacts your immunity, mental wellbeing, and risk of chronic disease—but not all sleep is created equal. You will learn about the physiological changes that occur during sleep and what makes for a truly restful night. Furthermore, you will gain strategies for improving sleep hygiene to ensure your cells get the rest they need.

- **Eliminating hidden toxins:** Your environment, food, and products expose you to various toxins. Still, your body has the ability to eliminate many of them as long as you are ensuring it is functioning optimally. So, while you learn the major toxic culprits and how they affect your DNA, cells, and chemical responses, you will also discover how to take advantage of your body's in-house toxin-removal systems.

- **Space as sanctuary:** Creating a healthy atmosphere at home and work is essential for your health. You will learn the science behind environmental aspects like natural light, nature, scents, and organization to reduce stress.

- **Emotional exploration:** Your emotional state contributes significantly to your physical health. You will learn the anatomy of happiness, how to build your emotional intelligence skills, and ways to optimize your "happy hormone" production. With this understanding, you will be better equipped to navigate your emotions and experience the benefit of living an intentional lifestyle.

◆ **Leveling up:** Your body likely needs some extra ingredients to achieve optimal cellular health—but maybe not the ones you think, and probably not as many as you assume. In this chapter, I will share the best natural ways to get the nutrients your body needs and how to use supplements to fill in the gaps.

Each chapter will end with a series of rituals which can help you put these concepts into practice, followed by reflection questions meant to help you engage with the content. After the reflection questions, you'll have a prompt to identify an action step you can take. These exercises help you build self-awareness and invite you to take ownership of your wellbeing. Therefore, I encourage you to engage with the prompts and be an active participant in your revitalization.

BECOMING THE WELLBEING DOCTOR

I can still remember that vivid experience in the morgue—one that changed my mind forever about how I wanted to work with patients.

When I arrived to work that Monday morning, a medical chart sat on my desk with a note: "An autopsy is waiting for you." I paged through the chart of "Mrs. Maggie" and wondered who had made the request.

After speaking with her physician and learning the circumstances surrounding her death, I agreed to perform the autopsy and prepared myself for the process. Before entering the cold morgue, I changed out of my green floral midi dress into scrubs, two pairs of gloves, booties, and a mask. As I stood over her chilled, rigid body, a sense of sadness overtook me.

With my clipboard in hand, I examined the outside of Mrs. Maggie's body. She had some old surgical scars and fresh bruises from attempts at resuscitation, as well as multiple IV catheters inserted in her arms and groin. I did a double-take to make sure this was the right person—her chart indicated she was forty-four years old, yet her body seemed decades older. As my examination progressed and I realized the full extent of her debilitation, I wondered what sort of life Mrs. Maggie had led. Had she succumbed to the notion that she was powerless over her health?

With my scalpel in hand, I made my first incision. One by one, I examined her organs. Her heart had three stents in it from a recent heart attack, her lungs were full of fluid, her kidneys and pancreas were shriveled, and her brain was atrophied. Every organ was measured, weighed, and examined, in search of a cause of death. The family wanted answers, the doctors wanted answers—and I wanted to give them answers.

On paper, Mrs. Maggie's death was a result of cardiopulmonary arrest, but her body had been failing her for some years prior to that. Several diseases ravaged her body, leaving her with a frail structure that would make anyone think she was eighty years old. In the following days, I examined the tissue from her organs under a microscope. Her cells were "angry," and they simply could not function any longer.

Her family was unhappy to hear about how each of her organs showed extensive damage. "Could this have been prevented?" they asked. It would have been insensitive for me to be so candid, but I wanted to tell them *YES*. We have so much more power over our bodies than we have been led to believe. I have now worked in a variety of contexts as a medical doctor—but in every context, this is a message that I wish patients understood more fully.

When I first started down my path to becoming a physician more than thirty years ago, my goal was to provide health and happiness to my patients and ultimately support their overall wellbeing. However, as I began practicing medicine, that goal quickly began to seem naïve. Instead, I would typically see patients in the emergency room, on the wards, then send them home based on their relative stability and hospital policies. After that, I would see them in follow-up clinic appointments. But something always felt off. I found myself taking the same notes about a patient month after month, with the patient failing to show significant improvements at subsequent appointments. My short appointments with patients and the symptom-management approach felt insufficient to help patients truly transform their health.

Later, I focused on pathology, a field in which I could diagnose the disease at the cellular level, which would enable patients to obtain the best possible treatment. Pathology is the study of disease's essential nature, especially of the structural and functional changes produced by it. Since I had a deep fascination with how the human body worked and how normal cells became abnormal, I obtained board certifications in Anatomic Pathology and Clinical Pathology. I also completed three fellowships in Cytopathology (from Weil Cornell), Breast, Bone, and Soft Tissue Cancer (from the University of Rochester), and a two-and-a-half-year fellowship in Integrative

Medicine (from the Andrew Weil Center for Integrative Medicine). Thus, I spent decades studying human anatomy on its microscopic, cellular, and chemical levels, learning everything I could to help patients truly transform their health.

After many years of diagnosing disease under the microscope, including more than one million cancers, I learned many factors affect our health. However, genetics is only a tiny part of the equation. The most overlooked aspect—one that is, for the most part, within our control—is our lifestyle.

> **#CellCare:** Lifestyle factors—what you eat, how you move your body, how well you sleep, and the state of your mind—are instrumental in determining the health of your cells, and ultimately your wellbeing.

Among other disciplines, I trained in mindfulness-based stress reduction (MBSR), yoga therapy, plant-based nutrition, culinary medicine, botanicals, supplements, and Ayurveda in my quest for answers. I have been privileged to share my knowledge on a variety of platforms as an author, speaker, and wellness expert. Since founding WELLKULÅ, I have been dedicated to educating practitioners and patients on how to restore cellular health and ultimately harness wellbeing. I am privileged to currently work and teach as the Wellbeing Doctor, a quintuple board-certified physician.

In my opinion, the information I share in this book should be common knowledge. People should know exactly how and why to take control of their health. Although all of this information is widely available, it's not always user-friendly. It can be confusing, and misinformation is abundant. Medical articles often have a narrow focus or can be frustratingly dense. In addition, I know that many people don't have an easy option to see an integrative and functional medicine physician. With this book, I hope to share some of the essential information that causes lightbulb moments for so many of my patients.

You might find yourself wishing you could simply download all this information into your mind, Matrix-style! Although that's not possible (I wish it were!), this book can be your reference guide until your path to wellbeing becomes second nature to you.

My goal remains from when I started my medical journey: I hope to see more people in the world live happier, healthier lives. After years of learning and practicing medicine, I have a clearer idea of how that will be accomplished than when I was a young medical student. I want people to understand that they have a fundamental part to play in their wellbeing: each of us has control over how much we move our body, what we put into our body, and our mindset. As a result, all of us have the potential to live in contentment with ourselves, in a state where we're effectively managing our health and happiness.

I've spent my life studying the anatomy of the human body. With this book, I've distilled the most relevant nuggets from my education and decades of patient work to provide you with *The Anatomy of Wellbeing*. This book is a global picture of how your body works, grounded in science-informed evidence. It's a whole-body blueprint for your health, happiness, and longevity.

So, where do we begin? We're going to start at the top—literally. Specifically, we're going to look at how your brain works and how you can activate your neuroplasticity for good. Your journey toward wellbeing begins with an understanding of how you can use rituals to rewire your brain and reclaim your health.

1

POWER OF RITUALS

"The way you use your mind is only a habit, and any habit can be changed if you want to do so."

~ LOUISE HAY, YOU CAN HEAL YOUR LIFE

"I FEEL ANXIOUS ALL THE TIME." MY PATIENT, ASHLEY, SAT across from me, trying to hold back tears. She had just been given a chronic illness diagnosis and didn't know how to manage it.

She told me she felt anxiety throughout the day, which was impacting her relationship with her kids, her marriage, and her ability to sleep at night. It bothered her that her physician had quickly prescribed medications for her symptoms without helping her get to the bottom of her issues. For instance, when she mentioned trouble sleeping, he prescribed Ambien; when she brought up joint pain, he told her to take ibuprofen. Ashley sought me out after feeling dissatisfied with her experience and explained she was looking for ways to heal her body from the inside out.

As I often do with my patients in our early sessions, I asked Ashley to describe her typical day, all twenty-four hours of it. Almost immediately, it became apparent that Ashley's morning routine was exacerbating—not helping—her anxiety. She explained that the first thing she did after waking up was ask Dr. Google questions about her symptoms. Then, she would read article after article, trying to figure out what was happening in her body. As a result, Ashley began her day bent over her screen, consuming information that increased her anxiety, rather than spending her time more intentionally.

"Let's start the morning with something purposeful and encouraging," I suggested. We came up with the idea of a morning walk. Ashley enjoyed walking and agreed that it would probably make her feel better.

It did. In addition to improving her blood flow, movement created endorphins and other beneficial chemicals, such as BDNF (brain-derived neurotrophic factor). As she got out into the sunshine, she not only got some vitamin D but also helped her natural circadian rhythm to align. As a result, she started sleeping better, her mood improved throughout the day, and her interactions with her family were more positive. She even made better choices with meals. Ashley once told me the morning walks gave her the motivation she needed to make positive decisions throughout the day. She was experiencing the ripple effect of one good ritual leading to another.

Ashley transformed her days by intentionally incorporating a purposeful, mindful task into her morning routine—something I would call a ritual. Instead of waking up and diving into internet searches, she chose to begin her day with an activity that helped her be more mindful, enabled her body to be healthier, and helped prevent her anxiety on a cellular level. She took the ritual to heart, too; she decided to leave her phone at home so that she could get in touch with nature and avoid the temptation of her mornings with Dr. Google. Even the act of planning her walk helped ease Ashley's anxiety. She often felt like many circumstances in her life were out of her control, but beginning each day in the same, healthy way inserted organization and structure into her routine, which felt calming.

Most of us fall into daily habits, whether those habits are helping us or not. Like Ashley, our routines may inadvertently attack our energy production from the very beginning of the day, inhibit our sleep, or set us up to feel anxious, as Ashley experienced. Some of those habits may even set us up for chronic disease.

We can do better than that. Through making small, deliberate shifts, we can increase our health and happiness and set ourselves up to embody wellbeing. That's the power of rituals. A ritual is a small, intentional, mindful change in your lifestyle that can transform your wellbeing.

HABITS | ROUTINES | RITUALS

When I ask my patients to describe a typical twenty-four-hour day in their life, they usually have a response at the ready. Most people find themselves falling into familiar daily rhythms built around key fixtures like their work schedule or school hours. We often begin our days the same way and end our days the same way. Familiarity is comforting and easy—however, these daily rhythms don't always help us. When we fall into rhythms that are thoughtless rather than intentional, we might be steadily moving toward dis-ease.

The word **habit** can describe these sorts of thoughtless rhythms. A habit is an automatic urge to do something triggered by a cue and often leads to a reward. The book *The Power of Habit,* by Charles Duhigg, describes this as a classic habit loop.[1] The loop starts with the cue, which triggers your brain to start the routine. After you execute the routine, you reward yourself. This begins to encode neural pathways that get stronger and stronger every time you complete the habit loop. It becomes increasingly difficult to get out of that loop, and you can get stuck.

For instance, you might have the habit of starting each morning with a cup of coffee. When you come into your kitchen every morning, you see your coffee maker: that's the cue. That triggers the habit of making your cup of coffee. Your reward, of course, is drinking the coffee.

A habit like this isn't so bad—but other habit cues might be. For example, imagine that one evening after getting home from work, you see your sofa. You're tired, and the sofa triggers your desire to sit down and relax. You turn on the TV as a reward, which tells your brain that this is a good habit. The next evening, you come home, see the sofa, turn on the TV, and experience that same hit of plea-surable dopamine. Soon, this has developed into a daily habit—but not a good one. That collapse onto your couch might feel good in the short term, but over time, this passive action can hurt your body and mind.

It can become tough to break out of a bad habit as your brain will always prompt you to look for the reward. Maybe you saw a McDonald's TV ad last night, and today you drive by one and think you should stop; there's your cue. So you go to the drive-through, order a meal, supersize it for added value, and there is your reward.

A McDonald's habit loop might give you a short-term reward, but it's going to compromise the function of your cells over time. When we fall into these habit loops without thinking about what they ultimately do for us, we can get stuck in rhythms that make us unhealthy.

No one starts out intending to be unhealthy—but when we thought-lessly fall into lousy habit loops, that's precisely what happens.

A **routine** is slightly better than a habit because it typically describes a deliberate practice. Brushing your teeth, taking a shower, making your bed—these are all routines that are implemented deliber-ately, with the understanding that they ultimately make life better. Routines can be helpful.

But they can also cause us to feel stuck. When people complain about "being in a routine," they usually mean it negatively. They might say, "I need to branch out of my meal routine," or complain, "It's just the same old routine, every day." Like habits, a routine can lead us to wellbeing or not. A negative routine will create a rhythm in your life that doesn't do much for your health or happiness. It may not correspond to what your life most needs; it's simply a prac-tice that you've gotten used to doing.

> **#CellCare:** *Habits* are for short-term pleasure; *routines* are for daily maintenance; *rituals* are for your long-term, functional wellbeing.

A **ritual** is an intentional practice that has a clear, designed purpose behind it. For example, you might engage in a ritual with the intent of healing your symptoms, improving at your job, or enhancing your relationships. Choosing to incorporate a ritual into your life is not done randomly; it's an intentional choice, prompted by a thoughtful, informed decision that will help you. It does not have short-term pleasure as its goal like a habit often does—although many rituals lead to a direct experience of gratification. Instead, the goal is global and long-term, taking in the bigger picture of what will lead to your wellbeing.

Whereas habits are something we do mindlessly and unintentionally and routines are something we do with a degree of awareness and intention, rituals are practiced with a high degree of self-awareness and intention.

HOW INTENTIONAL IS YOUR LIFESTYLE?

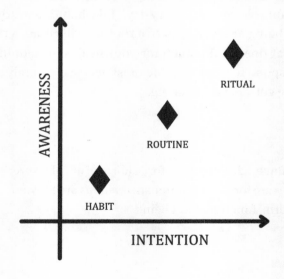

When you begin establishing these intentional practices in the rhythms of your life, they help organize your day. They optimize your daily routines in such a way that space is cleared in your brain to do other things. Take Ashley, for example. By replacing her Dr. Google habit with a morning walk, her new ritual freed up space in her brain to be present and mindful. As a result, she focused on being in nature instead of ruminating over anxiety-inducing articles. Ultimately, she came home ready to engage positively with her family. That was a good change.

Rituals can help you develop a deeper connection with yourself because they challenge you to think about what is truly important to you. You're asking yourself, "What are the most important needs for my body and mind?" Designing rituals reminds you that you have the power to take your life into your hands to make healthy changes. Whereas habit alludes to thoughtlessness and routines can imply complacency, a ritual is all about intent. It helps you identify an aim and a purpose; it invites you to do something consciously good for yourself.

That's why, for the most part, rituals are something you can look forward to doing. When Ashley started going for her morning walks, she quickly began to feel excited about starting her day that way and missed the walks when she didn't go. Because rituals are designed to help your body and your mind, the simple act of doing them will begin to feel like its own reward.

Throughout the rest of this book, I will invite you to consider lifestyle-related rituals that can enhance your wellbeing. Choose ones that sound fun. Put together a schedule for yourself that seems enjoyable. These are practices that you should want to do, that you *get* to do.

The concept of ritual has been around for thousands of years. Ancient rituals were often done to ward off disease, illness, or other opposing forces in the world. However, they aren't just good for warding off dis-ease; you can also use them to flourish and achieve your full potential.

It's not just our predecessors who believed in the power of rituals— modern-day brain scientists see their value too.

HARNESS YOUR NEUROPLASTICITY

Rituals do more than just transform your routines or set you up for success: they help rewire your brain. Neuroplasticity, also known as brain plasticity, is the ability of neuronal networks in the brain to change through growth and reorganization. In other words, the brain has the capacity to continue to evolve.

Scientists used to think that we were stuck with the mental habits and personality traits that we experienced as a child. However, deliberate neurological efforts, such as positive self-talk, actually cause structural and chemical changes. Furthermore, you can strengthen your brain's changes in either a healthy way or an unhealthy way. The first scientific evidence of anatomical brain plasticity came from research published by Marian Diamond of the University of California, Berkley. The study determined our brains have the capacity of both structural and functional neuroplasticity.[2] Ultimately, this means the brain can change with experience and improve with enrichment.

Here's how that works. If you are in a constant state of stress, your amygdala—the "fight or flight" part of your brain—has to work harder to continuously produce all the cortisol your body is signaling that it needs. This causes your amygdala to enlarge, and your prefrontal cortex—the part of your brain that makes rational decisions—responds by shrinking. Essentially, you've changed the structure of your brain.

If you change the structure of your brain, you also change its function. For instance, with a robust and enlarged amygdala and a smaller prefrontal cortex, your brain will produce more stress hormones and less frequently engage in calm, rational decision-making. So, you're more stressed out; you're less rational; your amygdala gets bigger; your prefrontal cortex gets smaller, and so on it goes.

However—it's not impossible to get out of this spiral, and rituals are one of the best ways to do it. Rituals maximize effectiveness by leveraging neuroplasticity. As the "plasticity" component of the word suggests, your brain is both strong and flexible. This means your brain can recognize new stimuli and grow appropriately; it can flex and change in response to new experiences. Rituals can give your brain the practice it needs to respond to stimuli in new ways, thereby affecting the network's structure and function in ways that promote wellbeing.

This is excellent news for anyone who feels stuck in a rut or suspects that they will never be able to change thought patterns or habits. Knowing that your brain has this flexibility allows you to take conscious steps to improve your wellbeing by activating your neuroplasticity. You have the power to change your brain.

#CellCare: The brain's structure and function can change as a result of experiences and environmental influences.

Here's how it works: when you do a specific action or think a particular thought, your brain creates a neural pathway, a kind of invisible circuit. At first, the path may not be very definite, just like you wouldn't see a distinct path walking through a field for the first time. But the path gets more established every time that action or thought is repeated. As a result, the connection between your brain cells gets reinforced and strengthened. This means that the pathway to that action or thought becomes faster and easier.

Think of a child learning to walk, for instance. When they begin walking, they frequently fall. But an adult can walk without even thinking about it because they've practiced so many times. Neuronal connections have been created in their brain to make the act of walking easier every time.

I couldn't do a yoga handstand the first time I tried—I kept falling over. But finally, an instructor stepped in and enabled me to do a handstand with his assistance. A successful handstand gave my body the chance to recognize how it feels to do a handstand properly: a neural pathway was formed. The next time I tried to do a handstand on my own, it got easier; the next time, even easier. Each time I tried, the neural connection was strengthened.

These connections get wired when we do any activity—when a baseball player swings at a baseball or a tennis player serves over the net, for instance. Those strengthened neural circuits help us form muscle memory until an action that once felt challenging becomes automatic. The same connections get formed with our emotions. Repeated thoughts and feelings can become deep and strong pathways in our minds. Sometimes, this can hinder our growth. As an example, if you constantly think negative thoughts, such as "The world is out to get me," you create stronger neural connections every time you experience that negative mindset (we will discuss this topic more in the next chapter).

Likewise, our influences can change the pathways in our brains for the better or for the worse. Putting yourself in a setting with people who share your views, for example, will strengthen your views. On one hand, if those people complain or otherwise serve as negative influences, you will probably adopt a highly negative mindset. (In fact, it's not uncommon for my patients to conclude that they would be better off if they took a break from the news, social media, or some of their friends for this reason.) Alternatively, if you deliberately surround yourself with people who are eager to learn, explore, grow, and evolve, you will eventually adopt that same positive outlook.

With an understanding of your brain's neuroplasticity, you can begin to rewire the destructive paths in your life. A constantly negative thought-life is not going to do anything for you. Instead, you can choose to start building connections that serve a purpose for your wellbeing. By the same token, you can train your mind to think thoughts that will promote wellbeing rather than ones that will harm it.

An intentionally chosen ritual can take the hand of an emotion or thought and walk it toward a self-controlled and calm place. It can help you identify specific actions that, when repeated, will change your brain and enable you to do things you've never done before. Then, when that ritual becomes a regular part of your day, these healthy practices will get easier, just like my yoga handstand got easier.

Repetition over time is a crucial component of neuroplasticity. These neural pathways are reinforced through repetitive use, meaning they will be shaped by whatever you do most of the time. For example, meditating once a month for an hour may not do much for you—but meditating for two minutes every day can make a noticeable shift in your ability to maintain focus and calm. Rituals are meant to help you build this daily repetition into your life so that you can rewire your brain toward greater wellbeing.

Most people have a sense of what it means to truly be *well*: it means you're healthy; you're happy; you feel positive, comfortable, and energized. If that's the goal, then the question becomes, how do we achieve that? Any positive change must first start with the *willingness* to change, which can be challenging.

STAGES OF CHANGE

As part of conducting a wellbeing assessment with my patients, I need to determine their stage of change. Changing behavior requires a multi-step process, and mental preparedness is usually required before those changes can be noticed. In order to make positive changes in your life through rituals, you must first acknowledge where you are at in your journey to change.

STAGES OF CHANGE

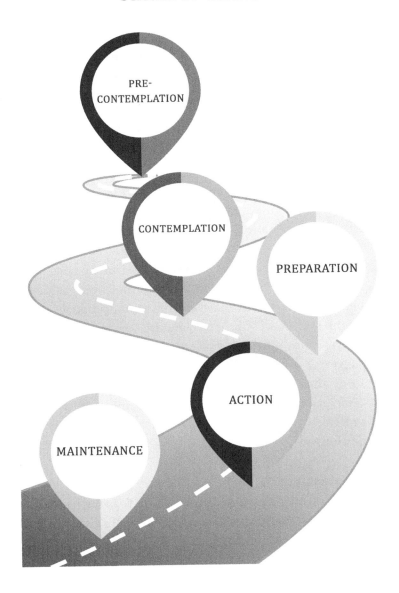

♦ **Pre-contemplation:** In this stage, change is something that you resist. You receive the information that perhaps you *should* make changes, but you don't want to deal with the hassle of implementing changes into your comfortable, familiar life. For example, a man might go to the doctor's office and receive news that he's pre-diabetic. The doctor tells him to change his diet and step up his exercise habits to prevent the onset of diabetes—but he doesn't want to.

♦ **Contemplation:** In the contemplation stage, your attitude becomes more ambivalent. You become aware of the pros and cons of making a change versus continuing as you have been. You know what the "right" thing to do would be, but you're still not ready to take action. Take the pre-diabetic patient, for example. In this stage, he might come home and tell his wife that he's pre-diabetic, knowing she'll insist he make some changes. He might still complain about making the changes, but his resistant attitude is beginning to contemplate the suggested change. These first two stages can go on for some time; people can often spend years in pre-contemplation and contemplation, pushing away change until their circumstances alter and they can't avoid it any longer.

♦ **Preparation:** In this phase, you accept that you need to make a change and actively prepare to bring it about. I often see people reach this stage when they start feeling physical pain or can no longer do what they want to do. For example, maybe the pre-diabetic patient realizes that his fingers and toes are tingling and hurting. The preparation stage is when he goes to his wife and doctor and says, "Okay, let's make a plan about how I can address this. I'm not feeling great."

◆ **Action:** This stage is when you start taking steps toward change. You're actively gathering information to help you learn more about the best way to implement that change. For our diabetic patient, the action stage may be going for daily bike rides and swapping out his morning bagel for a smoothie and multi-grain toast.

◆ **Maintenance:** The final stage of implementing change is the maintenance stage. In the maintenance stage, you do the hard work of *maintaining* the change through staying committed. This is no small challenge. For example, many people have experienced making a New Year's resolution that they kept up for three weeks before returning to their old habits. Rituals can be beneficial in the maintenance stage because they are purpose-driven, which helps you recall your commitment. Additionally, rituals are designed to be a lifestyle element that can be easily integrated into your day.

This book is primarily for people who have made it through the pre-contemplation and contemplation stages and are ready for the next steps. The following chapters will help you prepare for change, take action, and find ways to maintain change through incorporating new rituals.

Admittedly, it's hard to take the initiative. With so many distractions in everyday life, it is easy for us to let our minds and bodies run on autopilot, not paying attention to what is happening within us.

As you read the following chapters, particularly as you engage with the reflection questions at the end, allow yourself to register what is taking place in your body and mind. You may recognize, "Wow—this habit isn't good for my body—and this symptom is not normal." That is a positive realization because it can motivate you to connect with people who will help you recognize, refine, and maintain those changes. The process of taking the initiative and then pursuing your desired change will help you evolve—and that's a good thing.

Here's the goal: to experience small progress every day. If you want to become a better version of yourself, you need to wake up each morning with a willingness to grow, learn, and evolve. None of that can happen without a readiness to change.

> **#CellCare:** Making small, intentional progress every day will help make your cells strong and healthy so your whole body can thrive.

In the interest of implementing rituals as easily as possible, I will provide all the information you need to identify a clear purpose for that change, along with a path to help alleviate any fear of the unknown. Ideally, this will help you clear away resistance, go with the flow, and embrace healthy new rhythms in your life.

THE WAY WE PERFORM RITUALS

So, how does a person start to incorporate a ritual into their life?

First, identify the goal. We often start with a wellbeing assessment to identify the most beneficial areas for intentional rituals. That might be improving your physical wellbeing, decreasing your stress, increasing your energy, developing a better relationship with your spouse, losing weight, or pursuing more significant life satisfaction in general. The concept of rituals can feel broad until you identify a specific element of your lifestyle that would benefit from improvement. Next, determine the element that will experience the most significant impact from the small, intentional change rituals can provide. The reflection questions provided at the end of each chapter are there to help you identify these areas. Finally, we will use the momentum of your first chosen ritual to build onto a ripple effect.

Second, articulate your intention. The main difference between a *ritual* and a thoughtless habit or stale routine is in the naming of an intention. Having an intention gives you purpose, enables you to plan for effective change, and aligns you with your goals. Moreover, it will inspire you to put in the effort required to fully implement a new ritual.

For instance, I once worked with a patient who first told me that her goal was to lose weight. When I pressed her to think about her intention behind that goal—the deeper reason she wanted to lose weight—she said, "I want to lose weight so that I have more energy when I vacation with my husband. Whenever we go to Hawaii, he wants to hike, and I usually just stay in the hotel room. I want to go on that hike with him." When she articulated her intention, we

33

began to see the bigger reasons she wanted to work toward her goal: it wasn't just about her health and energy; it was also about strengthening her connection with her husband. Furthermore, articulating her intention enabled her to establish a clear reward and remind herself that all of her efforts were worthwhile.

Third, choose a ritual to work toward that goal. In my patient's case, who wanted more energy for her Hawaiian vacations, we now had a clear focus for selecting rituals to make her goal a reality. She decided that she would go for a ten-minute walk every morning. After doing that for a month, she increased her walk time to twenty minutes. She placed rituals *into* her life so that she could experience what she wanted *out* of her life.

Every chapter in this book examines a different lifestyle component, and each chapter ends with a selection of complementary rituals that may be used together or alone to better one's health. Decide what outcome you want, then select rituals that enable you to take steps in that direction.

We often tend to think too small when it comes to our wellbeing. We think, "I shouldn't eat that chocolate chip cookie," or "I need to bench press an extra twenty pounds." A thoughtful selection of rituals, however, invites you to consider your health on a higher, more global level. It may seem that small changes in your daily routine don't matter at first, but they have the potential to make a big difference over time.

Author James Clear gets at this idea in his book *Atomic Habits*.[3] He makes the point that small, consistent changes can ultimately lead to significant results. He recommends getting there through a concept called **habit stacking**. In other words, layer a new daily rhythm onto a habit already programmed into your life. For instance, if you have a habit of making a cup of coffee every morning, do five push-ups while the coffee is brewing. Or, if you have the regular habit of making dinner every evening, rather than watching TV as you prepare, check in with your child about their day at school.

> **#CellCare:** Incorporate new rituals using the strategy of *habit stacking:* layer a new intentional practice onto a preexisting habit.

What might this look like in real life? Here are a few examples.

Rituals in Practice

Annamarie is incredibly busy, but she has managed to carve out fifteen minutes to start out her day—and she makes those fifteen minutes count. For the first five minutes, she focuses on her mind with a guided meditation. In the next five minutes, she moves her body to her latest favorite song. In the final five minutes, she writes three things she's grateful for in her journal. This sets her up for an intentional day.

Yuki does meal prep every Sunday for her family: she starts by planning her meals, goes grocery shopping at the local farmer's market, slices all the fruits and vegetables for the week ahead, and organizes them in labeled glass containers. This advanced meal prep helps her and her family balance their hectic schedules with their energy needs.

I'll take a little more time to discuss Shane's story of developing helpful rituals to address his restless leg syndrome. Scientists haven't decisively determined the cause of restless leg syndrome, but it makes your body jerk at certain times of day and can be incredibly disruptive to sleep. Even though there's no definite cause, the syndrome has been associated with high levels of caffeine. I knew Shane was a coffee connoisseur. He *loved* his morning coffee, and I guessed he wouldn't take it well if I told him outright that he needed to decrease his coffee intake.

Instead, I asked him to write down how much coffee he was drinking. "Don't do any changes yet," I advised him. "Let's just build your understanding of what you're putting into your body. Then, when you get your venti lattes from Starbucks, look at the nutrition facts and write down how many milligrams of caffeine you're taking in. We want to shoot for less than 400 milligrams. Once we know how much caffeine you're consuming, we can figure out if there may be a correlation with the restless leg syndrome."

Shane recorded his coffee intake for a week and reported back to me. He said, "Wow—no wonder. I'm taking in over 2,000 milligrams of caffeine every day." That was almost certainly exacerbating the restless leg syndrome and may have played a role in other symptoms. I never even needed to recommend a specific reduction in his coffee habit; he came to that conclusion simply by being more mindful about what he was putting into his body.

We decided to cut his coffee intake in half, and he replaced the excess cups of coffee with herbal tea. He had the habit of drinking hot beverages throughout the day, so he used that habitual rhythm to incorporate an intentional ritual that served his body better than the excess coffee. Shane was so happy with the results that he took his coffee-drinking down to just one to two cups per day. He hasn't eliminated it in its entirety because he still enjoys the taste and the experience. However, his caffeine intake is now between 200 and 300 milligrams.

Shane's coffee habit was precisely that: a habit, one which he didn't think much about and one that gave him short-term rewards at the expense of his long-term health. However, when he built awareness around the factors behind his restless leg syndrome and sleep disturbances, he could use the habitual rhythms in his life to transform that habit into a ritual. Of course, he still wanted to keep his habit of drinking coffee, but now he's made it work better for his body by cutting back his intake and increasing his hydration.

If you already have habits in place, use the momentum you've already built to steer your daily rhythms in a more positive direction. For example, if you always had oatmeal for breakfast, use that habitual momentum to make the breakfast a little bit better. Instead of buying the oatmeal packets that are full of sugar and high-glycemic-index carbs, make your oatmeal with steel-cut oats for the week and see how you feel. Then, you can even layer on more nutrients that will serve your body, like berries and nuts— and then, wow! You will see how far you have come. These changes don't take much time, but your body definitely will thank you for them.

Remember that it's not just your morning routine that deserves your attention—it's vital to incorporate rituals throughout your day to keep it moving well. Wellbeing involves your *whole* life, which means using purposeful rhythms to optimize your *whole* day. Organizing your day with these intentional rituals will help you face challenges with resilience and calm. As James Clear explains, these small changes can make the most significant difference in the long run.[4]

FAMOUS RITUAL EMBRACERS

Rituals can help you achieve peak performance, so it's no surprise that some of the world's most outstanding achievers have rituals they are deeply committed to.

- **Serena Williams**, one of the world's greatest tennis players, has the ritual of wearing the same pair of socks throughout a tournament as long as she's winning. She also makes sure her family and friends sit in the same seats in her player's box for each game. The reassuring sight of knowing where each of her people sits provides a sense of comfort and support, along with a sense that everyone is in their proper place.

- **Rafael Nadal**, another tennis great, is famous for pre-court rituals. For example, he eats the same foods, in the same order, before every match. He also drinks water and recovery drinks in a specific order and places them in the exact same location by his player's chair. These rituals not only help his body stay energized and hydrated but also provide comfort and order, which helps him remain focused and prepared to meet the unpredictable factors of the match.

- **Oprah Winfrey**, talk show host, billionaire philanthropist, and influencer, starts her morning with twenty minutes of meditation. She says she does it because it provides her with hope, a sense of contentment, and deep joy. She follows the meditation with a treadmill session to get her heart pumping. Then, to wind down her day, she goes for an evening walk and listens to music.

- **Barack Obama**, 44th President of the United States, rises early (before 5:00 a.m.), about two hours before he has any scheduled appointment. However, he prioritizes getting morning exercise and never misses it.

- **Tony Robbins**, life and business strategist, author, and motivational speaker, uses a ritual called "Priming" where he incorporates three sets of Kapalbhati Pranayama breaths, an expression of gratitude, and prayer of guidance, help, and strength.

The more you understand rituals and where you can place them into your life, the more likely you will be able to live with ease when obstacles appear. Incorporating rituals is a flexible and doable process. They can help you rewire your brain to the point that healthy practices become easy and serve as the key to building momentum toward thriving, long-term health. Ultimately, they enable you to embody wellbeing.

THE BUFFER AGAINST UNCERTAINTY

Daily life can be full of uncertainties, stress, and anxiety—but rituals can serve as a buffer to all of that. When you weave daily rhythms throughout your day that are all purposely chosen to help you, you're more equipped to take on all of the chaos that life might toss your way. In addition, they can provide a sense of reassuring stability and steadily nourish your body, mind, and spirit as your life circumstances unfold.

Remember: life is composed of whatever you do *most* of the time, not *some* of the time. We are products of our lifestyles, and you have power over what that looks like. You have more agency than you realize in how you structure your lifestyle; you don't have to resign yourself to an existence that makes you anxious every day. You can choose to experience greater satisfaction in life (even without leaving your job!) and greater wellbeing in your body. As you begin to experience wellbeing in critical areas of your life, you start to enjoy your other experiences more, because your body feels better and so does your mind.

These intentional, small changes can help you reap the benefits of living a longer life. But it's one thing for me to say this. It's another thing for you to believe and act on it. That's why our next chapter will take a deeper dive into what's happening in your brain so that you have the tools to govern your stress response and embrace a mindset that can genuinely help you grow.

Reflect on Your #CellCare

Using these guiding questions, take a moment to build self-awareness and reflect on rituals in your life:

- ♦ How would you describe your typical twenty-four-hour day? In this average day, what kinds of habits and routines do you observe?

- ♦ When you wake up, how do you begin the day? What is your morning routine?

- ♦ As you wind down for the night, what is your evening routine?

- ♦ Are the rhythms of your daily life more a matter of habits, routines, or rituals?

- ♦ Are there any aspects of your daily routines that you think could be enhanced by layering intentional rituals for wellbeing?

DESIGN YOUR WELLBEING

In the space below, note your thoughts about where you might want to change up your routine with some intentional rituals in your day. Be specific. Write down your current habits & routines. Consider this a brain dump: a specific technique designed to declutter your mind and thoughts so you can organize your time and efforts.

2

TRANSFORMING YOUR MINDSET

I REMEMBER BEING IN SCHOOL WITH A FELLOW MEDICAL student, Yelena. We bonded over our shared love for cooking and traded recipes from our respective cultures: me, Indian, and she, Russian. But as I got to know Yelena better, I recognized that she seemed to be consistently in a negative mental space.

On Yelena's good days, she seemed okay—mainly because, on those days, her emotions were not disruptive to the other students in our cohort. However, on her bad days, her presence created a toxic environment. Whenever we were assigned a group lab project, Yelena always complained that she got the worst responsibilities or the most demanding tasks.

Although there was no truth to this, Yelena always seemed to feel that the world was against her. Instead of seeing her assignments as an opportunity to learn and strengthen her skills, her perception was that she was a victim of an unfair system.

That skewed perception created a lot of unnecessary difficulty in her life. It not only caused her to feel consistently stressed and burdened, but it also meant that she made the lives of all her fellow students more difficult. She wasted time trying to trade assignments, and she wasted energy complaining. The rest of us felt the constant cloud of her negativity, and any group project she was part of acquired a toxic atmosphere.

Yelena would vent to me that her studies were also hurting her marriage and relationship with her daughter. She often described various pains in her body that seemed uncharacteristic for a young, seemingly healthy woman. Once, Yelena told me that her parents raised her to view life as a competition to win. That competitive nature seemed to define her: Yelena experienced any moment when she was not "winning" as a crisis, exposing her deep insecurity. When she made a mistake—an inevitable experience for a medical student—she initially denied it and became combative. The correction didn't feel helpful to her; it felt like a personal attack.

Yelena was one of the first people I met with this kind of victim mindset, but she wasn't the last. Over the years, I've encountered others like her—patients, colleagues, bosses, people of all ages and cultural backgrounds. These were people who consistently struggled to achieve wellbeing in their lives. They all claimed that the problems they experienced resulted from some external circumstance—and, to be fair, perhaps that was sometimes the case. However, after extensive conversations and observation, it seemed that an internal struggle was often their biggest hurdle to overcome. Their negative mindset canceled their wellbeing.

THE ROLE OF MINDSET IN YOUR WELLBEING

Here's what I wish Yelena and all others like her knew: you are not stuck. You are not destined to remain the way you currently are, constantly struggling with the same problems. To assume that you are is to plant yourself in a *fixed mindset*. People with a fixed mindset generally believe this: "I know what I know. I know what I've learned, and I can't possibly learn anything more. And because of that, I also cannot be wrong." That fixed mindset assumes that you can't change. However, science shows that's simply not true.

Mindset is not a static thing; it is fluid. Our thoughts and experiences inform it, and it changes over time, just as our bodies change. Getting stuck in a certain mindset can impair your physical, emotional, and relational health; however, you can evolve through many challenges by embracing your capacity to learn.

Here's why this is important: if you're not open to the fact that you are capable of change, then you're not going to be able to change. By shifting your mindset, you will begin to realize you can redesign your life. Understanding these concepts will empower you to make small changes in the form of rituals, helping you get unstuck and reshaping your lifestyle and wellbeing.

How should we understand mindset? You can think of our mindset as the framework of beliefs that govern our thoughts. For example, an optimistic mindset operates with a belief system that trusts things will likely turn out well: "People will be pleased. I will succeed." On the other hand, a pessimistic mindset interprets information through a negative framework of beliefs: "This will go badly. I won't be able to achieve what I want. The other team will win." Our mindset, in other words, is our overall way of thinking. It's the lens through which we process our emotions and thoughts, which informs our general disposition.

You can have different mindsets about different things. For instance, you might have a certain mindset about the PTA at your child's school ("They always want something from me"), a mindset about your love interest ("They can do no wrong"), and a mindset about the political party you oppose ("They want to destroy the world"). As a result, you might respond to a piece of information in one way when that same bit of information would get a completely different response from someone else.

Your response, in other words, is what comes *out* of your mindset. Your thinking governs your behavior and informs your attitude. You can think of attitude as the emotional result of your mindset. For example, my acquaintance Yelena typically struggled with a negative attitude because she viewed most everything as a threat. But other classmates would come to the lab with positive attitudes, eager to learn and grow. They were operating with a growth mindset.

YOUR CURRENT STATE OF MIND

Your mindset is informed by many elements: your life experiences, the messaging you received growing up, your thoughts, and your cultivated efforts. That last point is critical: by positively reshaping your mindset, you can choose to experience the world with conscious intent. It might come as no surprise that there are pessimistic, optimistic, reactive, proactive, scarcity, and abundance mindsets, but they all tend to fall under a broader category of fixed and growth mindsets.

FIXED MINDSET VS. GROWTH MINDSET

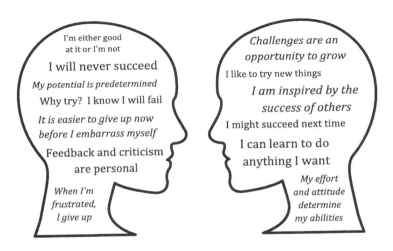

I'm either good at it or I'm not

I will never succeed

My potential is predetermined

Why try? I know I will fail

It is easier to give up now before I embarrass myself

Feedback and criticism are personal

When I'm frustrated, I give up

Challenges are an opportunity to grow

I like to try new things

I am inspired by the success of others

I might succeed next time

I can learn to do anything I want

My effort and attitude determine my abilities

A fixed mindset maintains the belief that you cannot change. You believe your qualities and abilities are *fixed*: if you are naturally good at something, you will always be good at it; if you are initially bad at something, you will always be bad. You believe that the way you were born is a good indicator of the way you'll live the rest of your life.

For example, imagine that a sixth grader has to do a certain number of pull-ups to pass a fitness test in physical education. The first day he is tested, he can't even do one. He might opt for one of two responses:

♦ "I suck. I can't do it. I'll never be able to do it. Exercise is dumb."

♦ "This is hard! But if I keep trying, I'll be able to do it. So, I'm going to practice, and in six weeks, I will dominate!"

The difference between giving up and going home versus trying and improving is all in mindset. For that sixth-grader, the fixed mindset is the one that says, "This sucks, I can't do it; I'm going home." And if that's the mindset that he chooses—well, he's probably right. He will go home, and he'll achieve a self-fulfilling prophecy.

What are other examples of a fixed mindset? If you were a late starter in kindergarten, you might assume that you will never have the ability to be a high academic achiever. If you struggled to get your first job, you might feel you will never come across new opportunities. Someone with a fixed mindset doesn't believe they have the power to change their circumstances.

There's a problem with where this assumption leads. If you believe that you have no power to change your circumstances, you are always looking outside of yourself to find happiness. With a fixed mindset, you will place massive importance on what other people think. You will constantly seek acceptance and approval, desiring external signs that will confirm your significance. For example, you might be obsessed with perfection when there's no such thing. If and when you fail to attain perfection in one of your goals, it will negatively impact your self-esteem. Like Yelena, many people with fixed mindsets take criticism personally and respond to it with combative behavior.

A fixed mindset impedes personal growth, happiness, and wellbeing. In addition, it can negatively impact your health and damage your relationships.

On the other hand, **a growth mindset holds the belief that you *can* change**. You're aware that you don't know everything, but that's okay—you believe that with time, energy, commitment, learning, and planning, you can get to where you want to be. Imagine the sixth-grader who takes on that pull-up bar as a challenge: "I can't do a pull-up today, but I'm going to be able to do it tomorrow!" That's a growth mindset.

As the name suggests, when you have a growth mindset, you are constantly growing. You view criticism as an opportunity to improve. You embrace challenges and are less concerned about making mistakes. Instead, you view the world through a lens of curiosity, looking to continually learn and evolve. This mindset is critical for making healthy and sustainable lifestyle changes.

> **#CellCare:** It's your thoughts that make you who you are, and only you can change the way you think.

A fixed mindset can manifest in several ways, but the ultimate effect is harmful in almost every variation. Similarly, the growth mindset is crucial for anyone who hopes to assert positive change in their lives in some form or another.

So, what conclusions can we draw from considering these mindsets? A negative *fixed mindset* can be detrimental to your wellbeing and prevent you from taking the steps necessary to improve your habits and health. Conversely, a positive *growth mindset* can help you make proactive decisions to improve your health and ultimately live a longer, happier life.

Remember: a *fixed* mindset is not something you're stuck with. A mindset is something you can *transform*. The rituals we will discuss in the conclusion of this chapter will help you reshape your mindset, leading to greater wellbeing.

#CellCare: The ability to transform your mindset and lifestyle is within your reach.

YOUR MINDSET CREATES OPPORTUNITY

People may seem to have a certain mindset by nature, but mindsets are not static; they change over time and are shaped by life experiences. If you're willing to embrace your capacity for change, you can grow through many challenging experiences. The last thing that you want is to stay stuck in a mindset that may negatively affect your physical, emotional, and interpersonal wellbeing.

Surrounding yourself with growth-minded people can powerfully influence your mental wellbeing. You may have heard the term *misery loves company*; this is the idea that miserable people find comfort in bringing people into their misery; in other terms, they have a fixed mindset. At the same time, someone with a growth mindset prefers to surround themselves with other people with this mindset. There is no jealousy here, only the thought that what is possible for this person is likely for me as well, if I continue to work toward it.

The idea of working toward a growth mindset might seem like a new trend, but actually, this practice is ancient. A *samskara* is a concept from Hinduism describing a mental imprint acquired from our thoughts, intentions, and experiences. Our mental impressions and actions are thought to play a huge role in our personalities and how we see the world. These can take both negative and positive forms. For example, a negative *samskara* might be, "I'll never be good enough." Over time, that negative message starts to inform your actions, behaviors, work, and interactions with others.

On the other hand, a positive *samskara* would be something like, "I'm always learning." This mental framework would, likewise, come to imprint itself deeply on the rest of your life. If this sounds familiar, you're right: it's akin to fixed versus growth mindset.

Positive *samskaras* can be embedded into your behavior with intention and discipline. Developing positive *samskaras* sometimes requires that you first recognize and catch negative *samskaras*, then deliberately think about the message you want to embed instead. You must approach this practice from a place of awareness. As you create neural networks through *samskaras*, you rewire your brain and form a new self-narrative. This practice can interrupt your stress response and create powerful opportunities for you to embody wellbeing.

Why should this matter so much? By maintaining a negative mindset, you set yourself up to experience constant stress, anxiety, and irritation. Over time, negative emotions accumulate in your body. Ultimately, this can manifest as physical pain in areas like your neck, shoulder, jaw, back, and hips. When you say, "I'm so stressed," you're probably referring to an emotional experience—but stress is a whole-body experience.

THIS IS YOUR BRAIN ON STRESS

Contrary to popular belief, stress can be beneficial for your body under certain circumstances. For instance, when our ancestors faced danger, the stress response caused the body to release hormones that increased blood flow to muscles such as the legs to enable fast running while decreasing blood flow to other organs such as the stomach for digestion. This effect is accomplished by **the sympathetic nervous system, which powers our stress response (also known as the fight or flight response),** allowing us to flee or fight like crazy in times of danger.

Here's how it works:

♦ The *autonomic nervous system* in your brain consists of the *sympathetic* and *parasympathetic nervous systems.* It coordinates almost all automatic functions in your body (blood flow, heart rate, digestion, etc.).

♦ When the *amygdala* in the brain receives the message that something stressful is happening...

♦ It sends a message to the *hypothalamus*, which activates the sympathetic nervous system, in turn signaling the...

♦ *Adrenal glands* to release a flood of hormones.

Let's pause for a moment to discuss your two adrenal glands further. The adrenal glands do more than just produce stress hormones. The *outer adrenal cortex* produces hormones that influence blood pressure and metabolism, as well as contribute to the production of sex hormones. The *inner adrenal medulla* produces hormones responsible for the physiologic characteristics of the stress response. What is the significance of this? Conditions like "adrenal fatigue" or "adrenal burnout" can appear with varying symptoms for people. As a result, because of its far-reaching effects, the treatment for stress may not be straightforward.

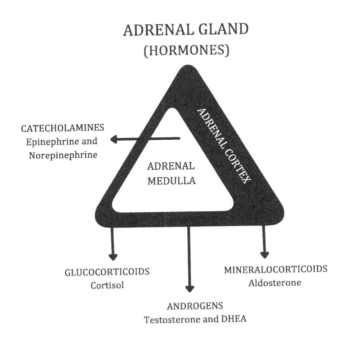

ADRENAL GLAND
(HORMONES)

CATECHOLAMINES
Epinephrine and
Norepinephrine

ADRENAL
MEDULLA

ADRENAL CORTEX

GLUCOCORTICOIDS
Cortisol

MINERALOCORTICOIDS
Aldosterone

ANDROGENS
Testosterone and DHEA

In modern times, there are still scenarios when this primitive stress response serves us well. If you're preparing to run a 5K, flee a fire, or play a championship tennis match up, you want all those stress hormones to flood your system. On the other hand, there are times when you would better serve yourself by functioning in a calm, level-headed manner, with lots of blood flowing to the brain.

Continuous stress can make it hard for you to function in everyday life since it prevents your mind from thinking clearly and your body from functioning effectively. When you are stressed, the *amygdala* in your brain is activated. Imagine for a second that the amygdala functions like a muscle, and every time you give it a workout by feeling stressed, the amygdala gets bigger and stronger. Essentially, that's what happens when you experience constant, intense stress: the amygdala becomes hyperactive and grows. When the amygdala increases in size, your prefrontal cortex, located at the front of your brain, *decreases* its gray matter. This results in a decreased ability to think clearly or effectively process your emotions. Unfortunately, this means that when you experience frequent, high levels of stress, you get increasingly *worse* at thinking clearly and calmly, and increasingly *better* at flying off the handle.

And it's not just your headspace that suffers from constant stress; your body also experiences significant harm. The continuous release of stress hormones can lead to suppression of the immune system, leading to chronic illnesses like high blood pressure, obesity, heart disease, and diabetes—just to name a few. Chronic stress hormones can trigger an inflammatory cascade, increasing inflammation in the body. Inflammation can attack your body in no shortage of ways, causing issues like joint pain, asthma, diabetes, cancer—and even mental health disorders.

#CellCare: *Inflammation* is the body's natural response to protect itself against harm. In an effort to heal, blood rushes to a wounded or damaged area of your body. This is helpful when you have an acute problem, like an injury or the flu, but constant inflammation triggers the release of chemicals that negatively impact your cellular health.

Stress can even create complications in your love life: chronic stress can seriously impact the male libido. Unfortunately, many men opt for the little blue pill to resolve this issue, but their bodies—and their love interests—would be better served in the long term by taking steps to reduce stress.

Chronic stress leads to a continuous release of chemicals, resulting in inflammation affecting the body as a whole. As illustrated in the graphic, your brain's pea-sized *hypothalamus* creates hormones that influence every part of your body. This structure serves as a control center within your body, helping you maintain homeostasis. When your body is chronically stressed, it can easily go out of balance. For instance, continuously releasing cortisol may interfere with testosterone and progesterone levels, ultimately affecting fertility and libido, amongst other things. Each of these hormones, influenced by the hypothalamus are closely intertwined with each other, impacting all of your cellular functions.

HYPOTHALAMIC HORMONE CONNECTION

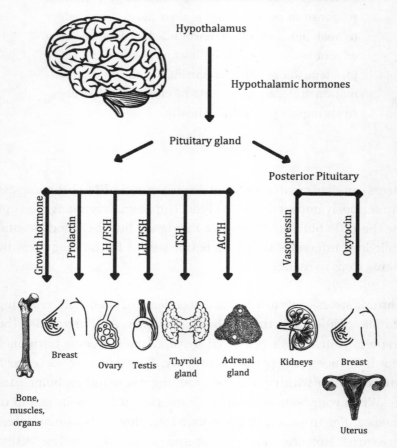

Given the enormous influence your brain exerts over the rest of your body, this is a critical area in which to pursue wellbeing.

Parasympathetic Protocol

One of the most important steps you can take to reduce the harmful effects of stress is to develop strategies that will help you regulate your response to stressful situations, moving you from the excitable sympathetic response to the calmer parasympathetic response.

In complement to the sympathetic nervous system, **the parasympathetic nervous system controls our rest and relaxation response**. Essentially, it helps our bodies return to a state of homeostasis, and we experience a degree of calm. We become creative, good at solving problems, and adept at managing difficult situations in this state. For all those reasons, we want to stay in a parasympathetic state for as long as possible.

> **#CellCare:** The vagus nerve is a key player in your body's parasympathetic response. It is the longest cranial nerve, extending from the brain to your gut, and controls body functions such as digestion, heart rate, and immune system. It sends messages to your body that it's time to destress and relax, resulting in improved mood, wellbeing, and resilience. You can use rituals to activate the vagus nerve (see "Vagus Nerve Activation").

Take the example of getting stuck in traffic. Suppose you don't have strategies to engage your parasympathetic state. In that case, your sympathetic nervous system might easily take the wheel when stuck in gridlock, flooding you with stress and anger. However, strapped in behind the wheel of your car, the stress response does you no good: all that blood flow to your limbs and away from your prefrontal cortex isn't going to help you drive any faster. Without regulating your system, you'll frequently experience a high degree of stress when driving, which means fight or flight hormones and chemicals are constantly released, causing damage to the body.

Even if traffic isn't a trigger for you, everyone has triggers that have the potential to push them into a constant sympathetic state. It's essential to learn your triggers and incorporate techniques to train your body to react in a parasympathetic state rather than a sympathetic one. You need to find ways to tell your body that you're no longer triggered and you're moving in a different direction. The more you can retrain your mind to slow down rather than react, the easier it will become to remain in a parasympathetic state. You create new neural pathways that help usher you from strong reactions and guide you toward a calm response. Your amygdala settles back down and your gray matter stays intact.

Stress can have a debilitating effect on the body, but incorporating mindset rituals can help curb those adverse effects. In addition, practicing these rituals can decrease your sympathetic or excitable state because rituals establish a sense of predictability—you know how you're going to respond, and you know that it will help you. We'll discuss mindset rituals that can help minimize your stress levels later in this chapter.

But before we do, you have another powerful tool at your disposal to counter the negative impacts of stress: *positive thinking.*

TRAIN YOUR MIND

If we can train our mindset to opt for a more positive response, we can help our bodies stay in the parasympathetic state. We become better at letting go of what we can't control, making the best of every situation, and generating ways to improve our situation. If we train ourselves to be positive thinkers, our brain and body will benefit.

And yes—training really is involved. Take pull-ups, for instance: every time you repeat the action of doing a pull-up, the neural connections in your body get more potent. This creates a stronger neural pathway that helps your body build muscle memory, meaning the actions that once felt hard become more accessible.

This can create a positive domino effect. As you strengthen the connection between neurons, you reinforce the action as a positive one: "Hey! This is getting easier! I don't hate this!" If you did three pull-ups successfully when you practiced, your brain now recognizes your potential to do three, and you will no longer put a cap on your future potential. You allow yourself to believe in your ability to do more, to take on greater challenges. The impact of this attitude is significant: research shows that optimistic people tend to be happier, less likely to participate in unhealthy behaviors, and more successful at work and in relationships.[1]

#CellCare: Health is 10 percent knowledge and 90 percent behavior.

Beyond simply increasing your potential and likelihood for happiness, positive thinking triggers biochemical and physiologic changes in your body that lead to beneficial results. For example, when you're thinking positively, you're in more of a parasympathetic state, meaning your thinking is clearer, and you make better decisions. Positive thinking also strengthens your immune system, making your body more capable of fighting off disease.[2] Positive thinking can also reduce anxiety, and positive self-talk can reduce negative thinking and false, intrusive thoughts.[3]

The converse is also true: negative thinking makes you more susceptible to illness. One study demonstrated that repetitive negative thinking was associated with cognitive decline, harmful protein deposits in the brain, and a greater risk of dementia.[4] Another study looked at over 100,000 women and found that those who were more pessimistic were more likely to have heart disease and had a higher chance of dying from it.[5] Keep in mind that your emotions have widespread effects on your body and its processes, including the release of hormones, metabolism, and immune function. For example, chronic low levels of cortisol over time from continuous stress make the body's immune system compromised, meaning your body is less able to fight the inflammation that ensues.

> **#CellCare:** Your brain is the most powerful organ in your body and requires its own kind of workout. Studies suggest that our cognitive functions decline as early as age thirty and that brain training games can improve executive function, working memory, and processing speed.[6]

So, how exactly can we begin to train our brains to think more positively? Through intentional practices that transform your mindset.

RITUALS TO TRANSFORM YOUR MINDSET

Let's take a look at some mindset practices that can help you foster change in your life. It is not necessary to perform all of these rituals simultaneously; choose one to try at first. As you integrate this daily rhythm and start to experience its benefits, you may consider layering in a second ritual.

Choose one ritual by considering:

- ◆ Which ritual would be easy to layer onto a daily habit that you already have in place?

- ◆ Which ritual will make the most significant difference in the wellbeing of your mindset?

- ◆ Which ritual sounds the most enjoyable?

Based on those considerations, choose from the following rituals to incorporate into your life. Feel free to get creative about how and when you practice them: you might do one before going to bed or when you're in line to pick up your kids from school. The more consistently you practice a ritual for a growth mindset, the more your actual brain structure and function will change. You can get yourself unstuck from an unhealthy fixed mindset to a more positive growth mindset by intentionally incorporating these steps.

Meditation

You can improve your emotional balance, self-awareness, and focus through mediation. But more than that, it changes your brain. A consistent meditation practice does the following:

◆ The *gray matter increases* in the brain, which causes positive structural changes in the **prefrontal cortex**. So, once again, our executive function can differentiate among conflicting thoughts, distinguish between good and bad, and make better decisions.

◆ The **corpus callosum**, the band of tissue that connects the left and right hemispheres of the brain and is linked with improved intellectual performance, *gets thicker*.[7]

◆ The **hippocampus**, which retains and consolidates memory, *increases* in size, meaning you have better focus and cognitive retention.

◆ The **amygdala**, which is responsible for fear, anger, and anxiety, *decreases* in size.

◆ In addition, numerous studies show that meditation relieves stress, anxiety, pain, depression, and insomnia and can improve attention span.[8]

Since meditation is an intentional practice (meaning it's not happening to you, you choose to perform it), it can improve your mindset by reminding you that you have control over your practice. Meditation isn't just something you should do when you're stressed or anxious, and it's also not something you can only do on a hilltop at sunrise. Meditation can be a regular practice, and there are even many different kinds to choose from. Here are just a few to consider.

♦ **Mantra meditation:** In mantra meditation, you repeat a word or phrase silently in your head, in alignment with your breath. A commonly used phrase is *"so hum,"* a Hindu mantra meaning "I am." As you inhale, you silently say "so," and as you exhale, you say "hum." This repetition is calming, but the purpose is not to stop your thoughts; it's to make you more comfortable observing your thoughts, yourself, and emotions. (Note: the modernized idea of "mantra," such as getting up in the morning and saying, "My body is a temple, I will keep my temple clean," is not the same as mantra meditation, but it can still create a subconscious shift in our beliefs, encouraging a growth mindset.)

♦ **Visualization:** This consists of mentally walking through specific positive images or listening to a recording of someone guiding you through visual images. For instance, if you have to deliver a speech, you can imagine yourself waking up, preparing for it, going on stage and doing well, receiving a positive response from the audience, and walking off stage. Then, mentally rehearse the experience in a calm space, so you have the sense of having done it already. This visualization can help simulate the feeling of what it's like to be on stage and experience success before you deliver the speech, making the actual event of giving the speech less stressful. You can do this many times over a period of weeks, and by the time you have to give the speech, your body thinks it already has. Someone can even guide you or provide a specific visualization when it comes to preparing for any situation.

♦ **Guided meditation:** This type of meditation can be done either with a recording or with a person guiding you through the spoken word. The goal of guided meditation is to activate your parasympathetic system, getting your mind and body to a calm space and into a deeper state of relaxation. The guided meditation can take you through an imaginary journey, but the guide might also use a more straightforward approach, simply guiding your breathing or providing you with a lesson for the day.

Mindfulness

Although the two words are often used in tandem these days, mindfulness and meditation are different. Mindfulness is about bringing awareness to whatever situation you're in or to what you're doing. It's not passive; it's an active choice to make our minds attentive to the present moment. Mindfulness is not the norm for most of us: a Harvard study found that we spend 47 percent of our waking hours thinking about something other than what we're doing.[9] For example, we might be watching TV but not necessarily paying attention to it. Or we're spending time with family, but we're thinking about work. Our minds are elsewhere.

Mindfulness seeks to correct this constant state of distraction by bringing awareness to a specific time and place. The same Harvard study found that people who were often distracted were less happy than those who were mindful. When the mind wanders, we're either thinking about the past or the future, and we're unable to enjoy the present. As a result, we experience happiness less frequently.

You can find ways to practice mindfulness throughout your daily life, such as the following exercises.

♦ One example is to use the **Five Senses** practice. In this example, when taking a shower, focus on your five senses: sight, sound, smell, taste, and touch. Watch the water coming out of the showerhead; hear the sound the water makes as it hits your body; smell the shampoo as you wash your hair; taste the water as it falls over your face and touches your skin as you bathe. The goal of heightening your awareness of all these sensations is to bring your mind fully into the present moment. This practice can be applied to any activity, from cooking to spending time with a loved one.

♦ Another mindfulness exercise is a **body scan**, which can help you become more attuned to your body sensations. You can do this while seated at your desk at work or lying down before you go to bed. Here's how it works: think deeply about how each part of your body feels, starting with the top of your head, moving down your shoulders, arms, body, all the way to the feet. Different sensations may be experienced as tightness, heat, pulsing, or tingling. Take your time and focus on one area of your body before moving on to the next. You're not necessarily doing this to identify if anything hurts, although this may occur during the body scan. This exercise is mainly to help you become more aware of the sensations of your body in the present moment, as our physical senses are tied to our emotional states. With practice, you will increase your ability to be mindful and fully present.

♦ **Progressive muscle relaxation** follows a similar pattern to the body scan above and can be an effective deep relaxation technique for insomnia, chronic pain, and anxiety. This practice requires you to tighten one muscle group at a time, followed by relaxation of that muscle group. Start by lying down in a comfortable position, inhaling and contracting one muscle group (starting with the calves) for five to ten seconds, then exhale and release the tension in that group. Relax for ten to twenty seconds, then move up the body to the next muscle group, maybe the hamstrings. Gradually work your way up the entire body, and as you release tension, imagine stress leaving your body.

Gratitude

Another mindset management practice you can incorporate into your life is the intentional expression of gratitude. You can do this any number of ways—expressing thanks out loud to loved ones, or writing it down on your own. By writing down the things you're grateful for, you help shape your mindset in a positive direction.

Consider **gratitude journaling** first thing in the morning or before going to bed at night. Here are some prompts you can use for your gratitude journaling:

◆ What is something I'm looking forward to today?

◆ What is a happy memory I have from today?

◆ Who are some of the people I am grateful for?

◆ What went well today?

Spending some time considering these prompts can help spark your "happy hormones" (i.e., the hormones that help you feel good, like serotonin, endorphins, oxytocin, and dopamine) as you create positive emotions within yourself.

Positive Ritual Tracker

Charting your progress toward your goals and the development of good rituals can also positively change your mindset. For example, you might use a running app to track your running times or take before and after pictures to chart your progress in a fitness or weight loss journey. You could also use a paper calendar or journal. Keeping track of your progress toward a goal can help you stay motivated in achieving it and validate your efforts.

Personally, I track five specific rituals I want to practice that align with a growth mindset. I write them down every week, examine the list, and check them off when complete. At the moment, my five rituals are gratitude, meditation, exercise, vitamins, and brain games. Then, based on my checkmarks, I can see how well I'm doing with my goals. I evaluate my progress at the end of the week before writing down the following week's rituals.

Many components of my day have become so ritualized for me that I don't have to write down the specifics. For instance, I eat ten fruits and vegetables per day, so I don't have to write and track that anymore. But when I started, I had to track it, as I was nowhere near where I am now. The key is to practice the rituals and be intentional about working toward them.

Journaling for Brain Hygiene

Journaling about your thoughts and experiences—what I sometimes think of as brain hygiene—can help self-reflection and acknowledgement of past mistakes. This brings self-awareness and enhances your ability to grow. Journaling can be a safe outlet, especially when going through a stressful experience. Some of the positive side effects of journaling include:

♦ Boosts immunity

♦ Lowers stress

♦ Improves mood

♦ Decreases anxiety

♦ Breaks the pattern of rumination

♦ Uses the rational left side of the brain to clarify thoughts

Research shows that journaling has positive effects on personal, emotional, and physical wellbeing. For example, studies have shown it allows you to heal from traumatic events, including surgery, quicker. In addition, one study examined the impact of a twelve-week positive effect journaling intervention on psychological distress and quality of life in general medical patients.[10] They found it may serve as an effective intervention for mitigating mental distress, increasing wellbeing, and enhancing physical functioning among medical patients.

Self-Affirmations

Affirmations consist of taking a negative thought and replacing it with a positive one. These can be helpful to do, mainly when those affirmations concern yourself. For instance, instead of looking in the mirror and thinking, "My thighs are gross. They have so much cellulite," affirm yourself with a thought like, "My legs are strong. I'm able to walk and hike and run with these legs." Affirmations restructure thought patterns in the brain and can transform how you view yourself. They can be done silently in your head, spoken out loud, or written down.

These affirmations can (and should) go beyond staring at yourself in the mirror and saying positive things. Instead, affirmations can be a process of thinking through your core values and reflecting upon them. This reflection helps you recognize when you encounter something that doesn't align with your values, equipping you to take on the challenge of overcoming it.

Breathe to Interrupt Stress

Imagine being stuck in a grocery store line when you need to get somewhere for an appointment. Your stress hormones build-up, you get angry, and by the time you arrive at your destination, you're frustrated, unfocused, and it takes you two hours to calm down.

Now, we know that may be beyond our control. There's nothing we can do to get it to move faster, but we *can* control how we respond to it. What if you managed to catch yourself getting stressed and interrupted that stress response by breathing deeply? The process of oxygenating your brain and blood can help you restore your body to a parasympathetic state.

#CellCare: You can't always control your circumstances, but you can control how you respond to them.

You can't meditate while driving, but you can choose a breathing technique like the **4-7-8 breath**: breathe in for four seconds, hold for seven seconds, then breathe out for eight seconds. Over time and with practice, a deep breathing exercise can decrease the stress response and help you achieve a more relaxed state. I'll discuss additional breathing rituals in Chapter Five.

Vagus Nerve Activation

One of the most effective ways to decrease your fight or flight response is by stimulating the *vagus nerve,* the long nerve that runs from your brain down to your abdomen. Here are some techniques to engage the vagus nerve and lower stress:

♦ Use your vocal cords: Creating a resonance or an echoing sound with singing, gargling, or chanting stimulates your vagus nerve so that your parasympathetic nervous system is engaged.

♦ Practice deep slow, belly breathing: Your mind processes one thing at a time, so by focusing on the rhythm of your breath, you can shift your focus away from the source of your stress. A slow and deliberate breathing pattern with a longer exhale at a rate of about six breaths per minute stimulates the vagus nerve.

♦ Generate positive emotions: Visualize what makes you happy, or better yet, do what makes you happy. Your vagal tone increases when you experience positive emotions.[11]

♦ Experience cold exposure: Acute cold exposure lowers your sympathetic response and increases parasympathetic activity through your vagus nerve. Consider ending your next shower with thirty seconds of cold water.

FROM ANXIOUS TO SELF-CONFIDENT

You can teach your mind and body how to thrive with disciplined parasympathetic states, using rituals to transform your mindset. By increasing gray matter, you will be able to think more clearly and with greater focus. You're more likely to engage in positive activities, which helps boost your "happy hormones." Your likelihood of achieving wellbeing increases when you are open to new experiences and stretch your potential. Furthermore, you boost your immune system, reducing your risk of chronic disease. Put simply: a growth mindset will enhance your overall wellbeing and cellular health. Incorporating the rituals in this chapter will provide a psychological safety net against stress and help you think with greater focus and positivity. A growth mindset enables you to live a longer, healthier life and allows you to devote more time to what you want to do.

If all of these benefits happen when you get your brain on board, just imagine what you can do for yourself by better understanding your body! In our next chapter, we're going to look at some of the foundational aspects of how your body works, starting with one of the smallest, most important, and most overlooked players: your cells.

Reflect on Your #CellCare

Using these guiding questions, take a moment to build self-awareness and reflect on mindset in your life:

- ◆ Do you often feel like you get the short end of the stick? Do you find excuses to avoid change?

- ◆ Do you often react on impulse? Do you actively try to make the best of every situation?

- ◆ Do you believe you are capable of making changes when they are in the best interest of your wellbeing?

- ◆ Do you think what you believe about yourself impacts your success or failure?

- ◆ Do you view challenges as learning opportunities, judgments, or criticisms?

- ◆ Taking all your responses into consideration, do you think you have a growth mindset or fixed mindset? Is this an area where you'd like to pursue change?

DESIGN YOUR WELLBEING

In the space below, note your thoughts about transforming your mindset. Then, write down a ritual you may want to incorporate into your life.

3

YOUR BODY'S
ECOSYSTEM

*"Eventually we'll realize that if we destroy the ecosystem,
we destroy ourselves."*

~ JONAS SALK, PHYSICIAN AND VIROLOGIST

EARLY IN MY CAREER AS A PHYSICIAN, I WORKED AS AN INTER-
nist. Despite enjoying the patient interaction, I was unable to
impact lives in the way I wanted to. I saw the same patients with the
same diseases repeatedly: heart disease, diabetes, high cholesterol,
and so on. I had fifteen brief minutes to meet with them, discuss
their symptoms, and prescribe medication. I knew that lifestyle
factors were making their diseases worse—but there was no time
for that discussion. Neither my patients nor I, as their physician,
were satisfied with the experience.

For this reason, I began studying diseases on a microscopic level as a pathologist. I diagnosed over a million cancers, observing the evolution of normal cells to abnormal cells. Compelled to get more answers, I started to study how lifestyle affects disease progression. For instance, how does an eighteen-year-old with no genetic predisposition for cancer end up with cancerous cells under my microscope? I looked deeper into the research about known lifestyle factors linked to cancer diagnoses, like obesity or environmental toxins. Many people assume disease is simply inevitable, and there's nothing we can do to avoid it. I didn't hold that view. A growing body of research was revealing a wealth of information on causation factors—they just weren't being applied to mainstream knowledge.

I would attend multidisciplinary tumor boards for different patients—these are conferences with a patient's healthcare team—an oncologist, surgeon, radiologist, pathologist, and others. We would discuss their drug regimens or the surgery they needed—but not what we could do to help the patient be compliant with treatment, support them emotionally, and *prevent* a recurrence. For example, we might be conferencing about a woman with hormonal-sensitive cancer, which I knew would be exacerbated by factors like alcohol consumption—but no one brought up the patient's habit of drinking two to three glasses of wine every night. I couldn't help thinking to myself, "If I was this woman and I was unknowingly doing something every night that had an impact on my cancer—*I would want to know about it.*"

It seemed we were missing a massive piece of the puzzle, and it was the same piece of the puzzle that had been missing during my fifteen-minute appointments as an internist: namely, *prevention*. I observed firsthand how cells could transition from normal to abnormal, and I felt that steps could be taken to prevent that transition—or to speed it up. Similar steps could be taken to restore cellular health for many chronic diseases. But even more importantly, I knew that people could prevent many illnesses before they ever started—by understanding the science.

> **#CellCare:** By tapping into what the research says is good for our bodies, people can prevent disease before it ever starts, enhance their wellbeing, increase their energy, and strengthen their mental and physical health.

Now, as an integrative and functional medicine physician, I have the time and scope to have these comprehensive conversations with my patients to reclaim their cellular health.

Here's a reality I've seen firsthand: having a disease is more painful and costly than preventing one, and prevention starts with #Cell-Care. Around 60 percent of adults suffer from at least one chronic condition, while 42 percent suffer from multiple.[1] So, if there's something you can do to prevent yourself from getting a chronic condition, or a way to drastically improve it—wouldn't you want to know about it? I know I would.

With that, we're about to geek out like tenth-grade biology nerds. Let's take a deep dive into examining the thirty-seven trillion cells that make up our body and determine our health.

THE ZONE OF FUNCTION

Think about a beautiful, pristine mountain lake—one along the lines of Lake Tahoe. The water is so clear that you can see to the bottom. It's a home to many species of wildlife, surrounded by lush vegetation, and adapts with seasonal changes. It's an exquisite ecosystem—a zone where everything is functioning optimally.

Now, imagine that Lake Tahoe is designated as the site of a new local dump. Within weeks, the pristine water is overflowing with garbage, refuse, and plastic. The wildlife starts to die. The plants, rooted in the lake's water, are poisoned. The whole ecosystem begins to deteriorate rapidly.

You can think of our bodies as ecosystems, almost like this lake. Similar to how animals, vegetation, and the land are all interconnected, *everything* in our bodies is connected. In the example of the lake, everything depends on the purity of the water. The water is the life force of that ecosystem, and when that life force is poisoned, everything connected to it suffers. Likewise, when we dump processed foods like sugary soda and fast food into our bodies, it's like a garbage truck dumping its load into a pristine mountain lake. Instead of giving our ecosystems what they need to thrive, we starve their ability to function.

In your body, that life force is composed of your cells—all thirty-seven trillion of them. Our lifestyle habits impact the health or deterioration of our cells, just as the garbage dumped into the lake turned it from pristine to a wasteland. When your cells are healthy, the ecosystem of your body is in its zone of optimal function. When your cells are damaged, your entire body will feel it. So when patients come to my office complaining about a lack of motivation, a low libido, or sleeping troubles, I tell them: "Your cells are *angry*. They need more support than you're giving them."

Within that thirty-seven trillion, there are many different types of cells creating tissues and organs. Let's look closer at what makes up a human cell.

Meet Your Cell

Cells are incredibly complex microscopic structures that make up a living organism. Think of your body like an iPhone—many minuscule pieces are working together to accomplish remarkable things, and all of those pieces need to function correctly for that biological magic to happen. I won't go into every element of a cell because, let's face it, I want you to stay awake. For our purposes, we'll look at just a few of the crucial components that make up these tiny, fascinating structures that collectively make up your entire body, in order to get a better understanding of how cellular health impacts wellbeing.

The **cell membrane** is a protective barrier, like an iPhone's case and screen. Not only does it protect all the other organelles within the cell, but it also allows molecular messages to pass *across* the membrane (like a touch screen) and specific molecules to enter the cell. When healthy, it keeps the bad stuff out and allows key nutrients in.

The **nucleus** contains our genetic material (DNA) and controls cell division; you can think of it as the iPhone's main computing logic board. Just as an iPhone's logic board controls basically all of its functions, the nucleus controls our cellular activities: it's what directs the cell to grow, metabolize, synthesize proteins, and

81

reproduce. When damage occurs, that damage is most visible in the nucleus, which appears differently than a nucleus in a healthy cell. Pathologists like me will most quickly identify precancerous cells by looking at the appearance of the nucleus. In the same way, if a cell phone's logic board is damaged, your screen will begin glitching, certain apps won't work, and so on. For all these reasons, the cell's nucleus is critical.

THE HUMAN CELL

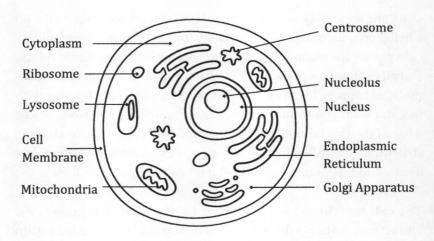

Another key organelle within every cell is the **mitochondria**, which is our storehouse of energy production. This would be like the cell's equivalent of an iPhone battery: the mitochondria are where *energy* (ATP) is produced. These tiny organelles also regulate our innate immunity, responding to pathogens by providing an immediate defense. Disturbances in mitochondria regulation are associated with diseases such as cancer.[2]

The **endoplasmic reticulum** (ER) is a labyrinth-like structure with many functions, including protein synthesis, lipid metabolism, and calcium storage. Under chronic stress, it can contribute signals that damage cells and result in metabolic disorders, such as age-associated disease, type 2 diabetes, and obesity.[3] We could compare this to an iPhone's processor, which runs all the apps.

The **Golgi apparatus** receives the proteins from the ER, which are then further processed to be sorted and transported to their destinations. This would be similar to an iPhone's RAM, which helps the processor run all the apps faster.

Why do we care about the makeup of a cell? Because collectively, these building blocks of life are responsible for countless processes in the body. Here are just a few examples of what cells do:

◆ Cells provide structure and support to the body.

◆ Cells are responsible for facilitating growth—your height, ability to build muscles, and maturation are all directly informed by your cellular activity.

◆ Cells utilize the nutrients from our food. They rejoice at spinach and balk at fast food.

◆ Cells are responsible for how we respond to external stimuli, like smells or hunger pangs. They alert you to eat when you're hungry, to jerk your hand away from something burning hot, to put a sweater on when you feel cold, and so on.

♦ Cells are also responsible for excretion; the reason your body sweats, cries, urinates, and defecates is all due to your healthy cellular activity.

> **#CellCare:** Every single thing your body does, feels, or experiences begins with your cells.

Actually, that's only the beginning. Different cells combine to form tissue that performs a specific function.

♦ **Epithelial tissue:** A group of cells that line the internal cavities and hollow organs, as well as the external surfaces of the body (skin)—ultimately *protecting* the body.

♦ **Nerve tissue:** Composed of cells that generate electrochemical signals and messages to *communicate* with different parts of the body.

♦ **Muscle tissue:** *Contracts* when excited to provide movement. Think of the heart or your limbs—both muscles, but different types.

♦ **Connective tissue:** Contains cells that *support* the body.

Most of our organs are composed of all four types of tissue. Take the stomach, for example. The stomach has a protective surface *epithelium* layer, called the mucosa, that absorbs nutrients and secretes enzymes. It has *nerves*, which send signals back and forth to the brain, like, "I'm hungry!" or "I'm full now." It has *muscle tissue*, which contracts to move your food through your digestive system. And everything is held together with the *connective tissue*.

Why is this important? When it comes to our bodies, it's essential to understand that nothing ever happens in isolation. Our cells and their interactions are *so* interconnected that everything we do affects how our cells behave. So, your lunch isn't just going to make an impression on your stomach; it will also impact your energy level, mood, immune system, sleep, and organ function—basically, everything!

> **#CellCare:** When it comes to your body, nothing happens in isolation. Our cells are constantly in communication with each other.

Once, right before doing a presentation, I overheard a woman tell her friend that she refused to give up her Cherry Cola addiction. Based on an earlier conversation with the same woman, I knew she struggled with fatigue, diabetes, and a hormonal imbalance. I shuddered when I heard her remark—all that high-fructose corn syrup was not helping her cells. Those Cherry Colas that she enjoyed so much were producing *more* damage in her body, making it harder for her body to beat disease and sabotaging her body's efforts to heal. In her mind, the habit was giving her a welcome boost during a stressful time. But as a physician, I had to wonder: Would she continue this habit if she understood?

Many of us struggle with this disconnect. We operate with a vague assumption of invincibility, thinking that our lifestyle choices won't affect our bodies—or, even if they do, that the impact will be small. That simply isn't true. Here's another example of how this disconnect might play out regularly in our lives. Imagine that a person goes out for a night of hard partying and heavy drinking. All that alcohol will burden that person's liver function. The next day, when that person wakes up with a brutal hangover, they'll pop three ibuprofen, further damaging the liver. By prioritizing short-term fun and symptom relief, they end up damaging one of their body's central systems of toxin removal. Eventually, the liver's compromised functioning means that person will feel sick and tired for much longer than if they were operating with a healthy liver.

And speaking of your liver, I think you might want a closer introduction to your essential organs. So many of us have only the vaguest idea of what our organs do for us every day, hour, minute, and second. We go through our daily motions, never considering the heroic efforts of our organs, but I want you to think about those things now. Seriously: these organs deserve a parade.

How Key Organs Function

All told, we have *seventy-eight* different organs in our bodies, each performing their bit of magic within our eleven organ systems. An organ system simply means that two or more organs work together to accomplish big things within our bodies. Take the digestive system, for instance—one which we'll spend a lot of time talking about in this book. The digestive system employs multiple organs, starting in the mouth. The esophagus gets the food down to the stomach, where it is processed in the small intestines with the help of the pancreas and biliary system. The broken-down nutrients then get passed on to the liver, the pancreas, and the gallbladder, creating enzymes and different hormones. The waste from the food then ultimately gets passed through our large intestine. The collaboration among all these organs makes up a single organ system, the digestive system. There are multiple systems just like this operating simultaneously, like a complex machine. It's incredible.

Next, let's discuss our five essential organs—the brain, heart, liver, lungs, and kidneys—which are *vital* for living.

The **brain** is the most complicated organ in our body. The central nervous system, composed of our brain and spinal cord, is responsible for all our thoughts, interpretation of external stimuli, and control of our body movements. Amazingly, our brain is never fully offline. It's always working, twenty-four hours a day. Even when we're sleeping, our brain is still doing something: it's sorting through all the information we absorbed during the day, storing what's important, and cleaning up the junk. Given the brain's incredible importance, we can be thankful that it's also the most resilient organ in our body.

That doesn't mean we should take it for granted, though; our brain deserves plenty of TLC. So how can we take care of our brain? Sleep, as mentioned, is undoubtedly an essential factor, but diet also matters. If you don't give the brain the food it needs or if you put a lot of unhealthy food into your body, you'll compromise the brain's ability to function at top form.

Many people would be surprised about the kind of food that our brains need. I've had people tell me before, "I eat healthy and I'm on a strict low-fat diet." Actually, the right kinds of fat are necessary for healthy brain functioning, since the brain is composed of 60 percent fat. No wonder so many people feel irritable when they diet! Granted, not every kind of fat will help the brain—saturated and trans fats don't support your body in any way, shape, or form. However, the *good fats*—foods with lots of omega-3 fatty acids—are brain food.

> **#CellCare:** When you take care of your brain, you improve your cognitive functioning and your mood. To support your brain, consider eating: avocados, olive oil, nuts, blueberries, turmeric, broccoli, pumpkin seeds, dark chocolate, and green tea.

The **heart** is one of the hardest working organs in the body: *every* other cell depends on the heart. The average heart beats about seventy times per minute (that's your pulse), and it pumps two thousand gallons of blood every day. Two thousand gallons! Our blood is truly our life force: it's what carries all the nutrients that fuel our other organs. Without the heart pumping nutrient-packed blood to our other organs, they're cut off from their supply and can't do what they need to.

> **#CellCare:** To strengthen your heart, exercise regularly, manage stress and blood pressure, and eat heart-healthy foods such as leafy greens, avocados, beans, and walnuts.

Incredibly, the **liver** is one of the largest organs in the body, about the size of a football, responsible for more than *five hundred* vital functions. What are those functions? Here's a list of just a few:

♦ Synthesizes hormones and proteins.

♦ Metabolizes fats, proteins, and carbohydrates.

♦ Makes enzymes and chemicals for other parts of the body.

♦ Stores vitamins, minerals, and glycogen.

♦ Produces the blood clotting factors we need to stop bleeding.

♦ Converts toxins into a form that can be excreted by the kidneys and bowels.

You can think of the liver as that unsung administrative assistant who does about a million different tasks every day and keeps everything in smooth working order. Given all the various responsibilities of the liver, you can understand why it would be so important to keep this organ healthy. Imagine how much harder your liver would have to work to do all its normal functions if things like medications or alcohol had compromised it. That would be like asking the hardworking administrative assistant to do everything while drunk. Unfortunately, our liver can't call in sick—which means it's our responsibility to help it stay healthy.

#CellCare: For a healthy liver, avoid fried foods, processed food, added salt and sugar, unnecessary medications, and excessive alcohol consumption. Cruciferous vegetables and citrus fruits will help protect cellular damage in your liver.

The **lungs** are the star of the respiratory system. With each inhale, the lungs move oxygen into our bloodstream, and with each exhale, they pull carbon dioxide out of the bloodstream. That's why the lungs are so closely related to the heart. Working as a team, the heart and lungs provide your body with the oxygenated blood it needs to function: the lungs deliver oxygen into the heart, and the heart then pumps that oxygenated blood to the rest of the body. Think of the lungs and the heart as ballroom dancers doing the waltz in harmony.

#CellCare: In order to keep your lungs happy, pay attention to the air quality in your surroundings, especially indoors. Improve the air quality in your home by adding plants or an air purifier. Thanks to its naturally occurring nitric oxide, beetroot juice can help increase oxygen levels in the blood—if you're not a fan of the earthy taste, make a smoothie out of it.

The last of our top five essential organs are the **kidneys**, which remove harmful toxins from the blood and transform the waste into urine. If you're thinking to yourself, "Wait—I thought that's what the liver did?" you're right, except the liver is higher on the corporate ladder, if you will. The liver is responsible for converting toxins into a form that our bodies can excrete; the kidneys then carry out that excretion process.

The kidneys' primary role is filtering fluids. They filter excess water and toxins into our bladder, which exit our body via our urine. That's not all the kidneys do, however: besides the fact that they're getting rid of body waste, they're also responsible for balancing the body's fluids, releasing hormones that regulate blood pressure, removing drugs from the body, and producing an active form of vitamin D. Technically, you can live with just one kidney. Still, that kidney would be more vulnerable to damage or becoming strained because it would be attempting to do double the work. Some of the warning signs that your kidneys are being taxed are high blood pressure and blood in the urine.

> **#CellCare:** The best thing you can do for your kidneys is hydrate, hydrate, hydrate—with water. Even mild dehydration can impair normal bodily functions.

Without any one of these five essential organs working properly, our bodies quickly deteriorate. However, it's worth mentioning the incredible importance of many of the other organs we haven't discussed—our stomach, colon, pancreas, reproductive organs, and so on. While we can technically live without these organs, they still perform unique functions necessary for us to truly thrive.

If you want your body to function at its optimal cellular health, you want your organs to function efficiently. It's challenging to be creative or operate with good energy if you're focused on disease, failing health, or pain. That's why implementing healthy rituals into your life can help direct the health of all these essential organs—and it's why so much of this book will be devoted to describing those rituals for wellbeing.

UNDERSTANDING YOUR DNA

There's another key element of your biology at work in your body's ecosystem: your DNA.

When I bring up DNA with my patients, some tell me that they heard about DNA from the movie *Jurassic Park*. In that movie, scientists "explain" how they took a drop of blood from the gut of a preserved prehistoric mosquito to clone the terrifying creatures you see in the movie. That's a fun theory—though not entirely accurate. Still, the cartoon illustration of a DNA strand from Jurassic Park is a fun visual for this significant bit of biology.

Your DNA is your blueprint for life. It contains all your genetic information. It's what determines what you look like—your hair color, eye color, height, and so on—but it also determines much more than that. Your DNA is responsible for how your body functions and how your cells might express certain diseases. For instance, your DNA might make you susceptible to diabetes. That doesn't necessarily mean you are guaranteed to get diabetes—but you might be vulnerable to it if your cells become damaged.

That's where *epigenetics* enters. Epigenetics refers to the influence of our environment and lifestyle factors in how our DNA is expressed. In other words, a healthy lifestyle, nourishing food, and a good environment can help prevent potential diseases housed in our DNA from getting turned "on." With a certain lifestyle, we have a chance to remain as healthy as our unique body can be. However, when lifestyle and environmental factors are poor, those bad genes can wake up, and disease can begin to manifest. To put things back in *Jurassic Park* terms, that's when the T-rex charges out of its pen.

You have no control over your DNA. This is because your DNA was assigned to you before you were ever born. However, you *do* have some control over epigenetic factors. That's why much of my approach with patients—and much of this book—is devoted to lifestyle factors.

The key to all of this—to healthy DNA—are those trillions of cells that make up your body. When your cells can't replicate the way they need to, your DNA becomes damaged, your organs can't function well, and your body suffers. So—how do you keep those cells happy?

SUBSTANCES FOR GOOD CELLULAR HEALTH

Much of this book will be devoted to acquainting you with the substances you need for good cellular health. In our body, cells divide and grow all the time. However, when cells are damaged, one of two things can happen:

1. First, the cell dies, and sometimes another cell will replace it.

2. Second, the cell alters, transforms, or mutates.

This second result is a scary one. When cells alter, they do not function the way they should in the body; therefore, the body does not perform its necessary processes. Worst case scenario, mutated cells become abnormal (dysplastic), which precedes cancer.

We can fight disease progress when we provide cells with the nutrients they need to replicate healthily. That doesn't just mean eating the right foods—although that's a big part of it. It also entails guarding against environmental toxins and caring for your body through practices like movement and restful sleep. It requires a whole-body approach.

But it's not just disease you should be thinking about when caring for your body—it's *thriving* that is the ultimate goal. Unfortunately, none of us can achieve wellbeing when we're tired, irritable, moody, or sick. That's why you must combat the epidemic of *dis-ease*. In order to be at the peak of your cellular health, every one of your cells needs to be able to function with *ease* to enable your body to function at its best.

So, what are some of the specific substances that your body needs for good cellular health? When I do preliminary tests with my patients, I look at a breakdown of their antioxidants, vitamins, minerals, amino acids, toxin burden, and other key metabolites. If all of these ingredients were listed on a menu that you showed to your cells, they would say, "Yes, I want *all of them.*" These are the elements that keep them happy, healthy, and thriving.

Antioxidants

Antioxidants are molecules that fight free radicals in your body. Free radicals are unstable atoms that damage cells, leading to oxidative stress, ultimately causing disease.[4] Oxidative stress results from the imbalance between the production of free radicals and the body's ability to eliminate them or repair the damage with antioxidants. For this reason, it's important to supply these substances to the cells to reduce oxidative stress.

There are several factors that contribute to oxidative stress, including inflammation, environmental toxins, and a diet high in sugar, fat and alcohol. The body's ability to combat free radicals diminishes with age, which is why it's so crucial to take good care of your cells from an early age.

What are the consequences of oxidative stress? Many! Oxidative stress is linked to central nervous system diseases such as Alzheimer's and dementia,[5] autoimmune and inflammatory disorders,[6] age-related appearance changes, cancer, and much more. Antioxidants play a role in fighting these disease-causing agents, and the best source for them is your food. The antioxidants listed below all work to fight free radicals, but they also perform other important jobs.

Key Antioxidants

♦ **Vitamin A:** Important for immune functioning, vision, healthy cell growth, and gene expression. Insufficient vitamin A can impair immunity and tissue regeneration and increase infections. Orange-colored foods, such as sweet potatoes, carrots, pumpkin, and butternut squash, contain carotenoid compounds that are converted into vitamin A. Dark leafy greens, such as spinach and kale, are also good sources.

♦ **Vitamin C:** Aids in regeneration of antioxidants, synthesizes collagen (which makes skin firmer), is necessary for immune functioning (helps produce white blood cells and antibodies), and participates in cholesterol metabolism. Vitamin C deficiency can affect your oral health, immunity, and contribute to fatigue and irritability. Sources of vitamin C include oranges, strawberries, sweet red peppers, broccoli, and tomatoes.

♦ **Vitamin E:** Influences immune functioning, regulates cell signals, and is important to maintain healthy hair, skin, and nails. Insufficient vitamin E levels can lead to muscle pain or weakness, oxidative damage of the skin, and cognitive impairment. Sources include carrots, avocados, dark leafy greens, nuts, and seeds.

♦ **CoQ10:** A powerful antioxidant made in the body and stored in cell membranes, it is essential for energy production and pH regulation in the body. Insufficient levels of CoQ10 can aggravate inflammation, oxidative stress, cancer, and other diseases. Sources include whole grains, nuts (sesame seeds, pistachios), vegetables (spinach, cauliflower, broccoli), and fruits (oranges, strawberries).

♦ **Alpha-Lipoic Acid:** Important for energy production, antioxidant activity, and insulin signaling. Good levels of Alpha-Lipoic Acid can improve the way our body uses sugar and protect against age-related cognitive decline. Sources include spinach, broccoli, tomatoes, peas, and Brussels sprouts.

♦ **Glutathione:** Important in antioxidant activity and detoxification. Deficiency may result in impaired detoxification, altered immunity, and increased risk of chronic disease. Our need for glutathione increases with high-fat diets, smoking, alcohol, and toxic exposures. Sources include sulfur-rich foods (broccoli, watercress, cauliflower), allium vegetables (garlic, shallots, onions), Brazil nuts, spinach, avocados, asparagus, and okra. The body does not fully absorb dietary glutathione, but you can help decrease oxidative stress with these foods.

B Vitamins

B vitamins are a group of eight nutrients that boost your energy. In fact, if you chose to take B vitamins in the morning, you would get a boost of energy without ever needing caffeine. Many of the cellular processes I'm about to describe are associated with energy production, making B vitamins particularly important.

KEY B VITAMINS

♦ **Thiamin (B1):** An essential cofactor for enzymes synthesizing energy (ATP) from food and making DNA. Insufficient levels can lead to fatigue, irritability, nerve damage, blurry vision, and inability to think clearly. Sources include whole grains, lentils, spinach, and peas.

♦ **Riboflavin (B2):** Plays a vital role in maintaining the body's energy supply, detoxification, and antioxidant function. Low B2 levels can lead to low energy by causing mitochondrial dysfunction and oxidative stress. Sources include cruciferous vegetables, asparagus, spinach, mushrooms, sweet potatoes, and whole grains.

♦ **Niacin (B3):** Supports energy production, eases arthritis, and boosts brain function; important for making fatty acids, cholesterol synthesis, and DNA repair. Insufficient levels of B3 can be associated with depression, memory loss, dementia, fatigue, and diarrhea. Sources include whole grains, peanuts, seeds, and lentils.

♦ **Pantothenic acid (B5):** Helps produce energy by breaking down fats and carbohydrates; promotes healthy skin, hair, eyes, and liver; keeps your digestive tract healthy and makes stress- and sex-related hormones in the adrenal glands. Insufficient amounts may lead to tiredness, depression, irritability, sleep disorders, and muscle cramps. Sources include lentils, soybeans, split peas, mushrooms, avocados, broccoli, sweet potatoes, and cabbage.

♦ **Pyridoxine (B6):** Important for our neurotrans-mitters (serotonin and dopamine) and the synthe-sis of hemoglobin, which makes our red blood cells. Insufficient levels of B6 can lead to neurological symptoms like irritability, depression, impaired immunity, and other mental health disorders. Sources include whole grains, soybeans, chickpeas, lentils, nuts, seeds, and spinach.

♦ **Biotin (B7):** Important in DNA replication and transcription and fatty acid synthesis. Low levels of B7 can result in impaired immunity, hair loss, and depression. Sources include whole grains, nuts, sunflower seeds, avocados, and sweet potatoes.

♦ **Folate (B9):** Plays a crucial role in making DNA and red blood cells. Low levels may result in fatigue, impaired immunity, heart disease, birth defects, and increased cancer risk. Sources include green vegetables, beans, legumes, and fortified grains.

♦ **Cobalamin (B12):** Important for energy production, making red blood cells, and maintaining nerve cells. Insufficient levels of B12 can cause neurologic symptoms like memory loss, depression, and dementia. Sources include nutritional yeast, fortified cereals, chlorella, and Nori seaweed.

Note all the previously mentioned antioxidants and vitamins can be compromised by excessive alcohol intake and several medications, including antibiotics, oral contraceptives, tricyclic antidepressants, and many more.

Minerals

Our body needs not only vitamins and antioxidants but also minerals. Minerals are elements found in our food that are required to support our body to function normally. These include potassium, sodium, chloride, iron, zinc, iodine, copper, manganese, selenium, molybdenum, chromium, and magnesium. We will discuss just a few in detail.

KEY MINERALS

♦ **Magnesium:** Involved in more than three hundred metabolic reactions in the body, including cell signaling. Many people are low in magnesium because our soil is depleted of it, and it's not as prevalent in our food supply as it was in the past. Low levels can result in constipation, depression, and muscle weakness. Sources include pumpkin seeds, dark leafy greens, chocolate, and nuts.

♦ **Manganese:** Important for bone and cartilage formation, digestion, antioxidant function, and energy production. Insufficient amounts can affect inflammation, oxidative stress, infertility, and many other things. Sources include whole grains, legumes, and dark leafy greens.

♦ **Zinc:** Important for immunity, reproduction, and digestion. Insufficient zinc levels can lead to hair loss and difficulty in healing from various impairments. Sources include soybeans, nuts, pumpkin seeds, and root vegetables.

♦ **Molybdenum:** Cofactor in some cellular processes to help metabolize toxins. Insufficient levels can result in neurological disorders. Sources include nuts, beans, and lentils.

Amino Acids

We have twenty amino acids in our bodies, and all are important, but nine are considered essential. So, what do amino acids do? They are the building blocks that make up proteins and hormones, which affect nearly all our bodily functions. Our bodies can internally make eleven of them, but the nine essential amino acids must be absorbed through food.

When you're eating a nutritionally poor, undiversified diet, you may be missing some of these amino acids. That deficiency will cause problems with neurotransmitter and hormone production. For instance, you might not be able to make serotonin (the "feel-good" hormone) or you may struggle to produce enough melatonin to help you fall asleep. However, a nutrient-rich diet can help you get the amino acids you need for good cellular health. I've provided some examples of foods that are good sources for your essential amino acids in the box below. This list is not complete, but it demonstrates the variety of foods we need to eat in order to help our body function well.

NINE ESSENTIAL AMINO ACIDS

♦ **Histidine:** Used to produce histamine, a neurotransmitter vital to immune response, digestion, sexual function, and sleep–wake cycles. It also helps protect you from damage caused by heavy metals and radiation. Sources include tofu, pumpkin seeds, navy beans, and peanut butter.

♦ **Isoleucine:** Involved in muscle metabolism, immune function, hemoglobin production, and energy regulation. Sources include tofu, lentils, whole grains, nuts, seeds, and beans.

♦ **Leucine:** Involved in muscle growth and helps prevent muscle deterioration with age. Sources include tofu, pumpkin seeds, and navy beans.

♦ **Lysine:** Plays a role in protein, hormone enzyme, and energy production. It also helps with immune function and the production of collagen and elastin. Sources include soybeans, tofu, beans, and green peas.

♦ **Methionine:** Important for tissue growth, absorption of zinc and selenium, and detoxification. It may also help reduce cholesterol levels and damage from heavy metals. Sources include tofu, sweet potatoes, avocados, whole grains, and quinoa.

- **Phenylalanine:** Important in creating brain signaling molecules such as dopamine, norepinephrine, and epinephrine. Sources include avocados, sweet potatoes, mushrooms, bananas, and dried coconut.

- **Threonine:** Helps the liver properly regulate fat metabolism and is essential to collagen, elastin, and digestive enzyme production. Sources include green peas, pumpkin seeds, edamame, and tofu.

- **Tryptophan:** Necessary for sleep, mood, and appetite regulation. It also produces niacin, which is essential in creating the neurotransmitter serotonin. Sources include peanuts, pumpkin seeds, sesame seeds, and soy.

- **Valine:** Helps stimulate muscle growth and regeneration and is important in energy production. Sources include tofu, pumpkin seeds, hemp seeds, pistachios, flax seeds, oatmeal, and broccoli.

Other Important Vitamins

We have already covered vitamins A and E; now let's talk about the remaining fat soluble vitamins D and K.

THESE ARE ESSENTIAL, TOO

♦ **Vitamin D:** Crucial for immune health, bone health, and cancer prevention. The sun is a natural source of vitamin D, but many people still remain deficient. A person living in the northern hemisphere, people of color, and exclusively breastfed babies can be deficient in vitamin D. The good news is deficiencies can be improved through diet and supplementation. Plant-based sources include fortified soy milk, almond milk or rice milk, and mushrooms (maitake, morel, oyster, and shiitake).

♦ **Vitamin K:** Important for bone and heart health, as well as blood clotting. Sources include dark leafy greens (kale, mustard greens, Swiss chard, collard green, spinach), broccoli, and Brussels sprouts.

In reading about all these key ingredients for cellular health, your first instinct might be to run to the nearest drug store and load up your cart with supplements. But let me give you some advice—don't.

Simply taking a vitamin is not going to solve the problem—in fact, playing fast and loose with supplements without first getting a doctor's advice can create problems. This is because when you take a vitamin, your body does not necessarily absorb all of it. For example, if you have ever taken a B vitamin, you might notice that your pee turns a bright yellow color. That's because half of the B vitamin is getting peed out, rather than absorbed. There's a stability factor also: we're meant to take in vitamins naturally from foods, which provide stabilizing factors. If you try to get all your key cellular ingredients from supplements, you're missing plant-based elements that help with this stabilization, like phytonutrients (more on that later).

The best source for all these ingredients is a diversified whole food diet. Scientists and doctors are still learning why our bodies tend to absorb nutrients better from food than supplements. However, those whole foods do something good for our bodies that we can't get from pills.

What's the point in discussing all these antioxidant and vitamin-rich foods? So that you can really take a look at whether you are giving your cells what they need to thrive. Imagine trying to grow a garden, but never watering or fertilizing your plants. The plants would be weak and small, or may not even survive. The same effect happens when you deprive your cells of needed nutrients—only they don't only die; sometimes they mutate into something worse, like cancerous cells or chronic disease.

This chapter sought to help you *understand* some the substances your body needs for good cellular health. Now that the groundwork has been established, the following chapters will help you put this knowledge into action with rituals for wellbeing.

FLOURISH

Understanding the delicate ecosystem that is your body lays the groundwork for all of our other content. If one ingredient is missing, you're not going to be able to operate at optimal cellular health. Everything your body feels and experiences relates to your cellular health. That means every step that you take to make your cells healthier will help your body work better. Everything is interconnected. Each system and cell in your body relies on the others functioning well.

While it's true our bodies have a fantastic ability to bounce back, many of us are making it incredibly difficult for our bodies to do so. That's why so many older people are heavily dependent on medications to cope with their varied symptoms of compromised health. In this current day and age, we see some of the most extended lifespans in history—at least, if you're evaluating age according to the number of years. However, we do not have a longer *healthspan*. We're not healthier just because we're living longer. We live longer because a cornucopia of medications keeps us alive.

But to truly live—to thrive and experience health, well into our old age—we need to care for our health right where it starts. Consequently, the remainder of this book will explore the anatomy of wellbeing: how our lifestyle choices can damage our cells or help these building blocks of life genuinely flourish. You may have noticed at several points throughout this chapter that the food you eat plays a *huge* role in your #CellCare, which is why our next stop is Culinary Nourishment.

Reflect on Your #CellCare

Using these guiding questions, take a moment to build self-awareness and reflect on #CellCare in your life:

♦ Are you able to recognize when your body's functioning isn't optimal?

♦ Have you been experiencing persistent, ongoing symptoms (gut issues, migraines, unexplained fatigue, etc.) and doctors have not been able to diagnose the problem?

♦ Are there days when your usual tasks become more difficult for no apparent reason?

♦ What is your regular routine for supporting your cells, tissues, and organs?

♦ Is your current diet rich in antioxidants, vitamins, and minerals?

DESIGN YOUR WELLBEING

In the space below, note some of your key takeaways about what nutrients your body needs. Then, over the next week, take inventory of the variety of foods and supplements you currently consume and how they make you feel. Is there somewhere you could make some changes? If so, write it down here.

4

CULINARY NOURISHMENT

"All disease begins in the gut."

~ HIPPOCRATES

LIAM, A FORTY-YEAR-OLD FINANCIAL ADVISOR, CAME TO SEE me because he wanted to explore a new approach to his health. He enjoyed dinner parties on the weekends, business meetings over burgers, and drinking beer with his fantasy football team. At our first meeting, Liam told me he used to eat and drink whatever he wanted but now felt fatigued and worn out the next day. He was having trouble keeping up with his toddler, and his wife mentioned his recent weight gain in their holiday photo. In addition, blood tests from his family physician revealed an increase in his cholesterol level, which surprised him and made him feel disappointed with himself. In addition, his sleep and libido were impacted, prompting him to take medication. Liam was at a loss and did not want to be on lifelong prescriptions. Rather, he wanted me to help him naturally lower his cholesterol, lose weight, and optimize his health.

I talked with Liam on the phone before our first meeting, and he told me he was "pretty buff." He'd been doing weight training work-outs five days a week and chugging protein shakes before and after working out. However, after his physical exam and a review of his blood work, it was clear that Liam was not as healthy as he wanted to believe. The most interesting thing about our appointment was what happened immediately afterward: I saw him drive away, park his car at the steakhouse across the street, and go in!

I could tell that Liam's health challenges resulted from what he was putting into his body—the beer, the steak, and all the excess protein. So, I asked him to meet me at a grocery store for our next appoint-ment to better understand what sorts of foods he liked and what he was purchasing. Liam was the cook in the family, so this was not such a far-fetched idea for him to go to the store.

At the grocery store, Liam showed me what he typically bought. He walked right past the fresh produce and went straight to the frozen foods aisle. He picked up a couple of frozen pizzas, burgers, and chicken. Once we got out of the frozen aisle, Liam made his way over to the butchery, where he proceeded to add a half-pound of ham, provolone cheese, and turkey. I could see he was into any available meat! I thought, "No wonder Liam is having issues with his choles-terol." With animal protein being high in saturated fat, his diet was not good for his cardiovascular health, nor was it well balanced. That shopping cart was devoid of anything green—no vegetable in sight, except for the five-pound bag of russet potatoes.

After my analysis, I concluded that Liam had metabolic syndrome, a cluster of conditions increasing one's risk of heart disease, stroke, and type 2 diabetes. Metabolic syndrome makes losing weight a struggle, which explained why the other men at Liam's gym were losing weight, but he was not. Also, Liam hadn't yet connected his diet and his disappointing performance in the bedroom. Obesity and increased insulin levels suppress sex hormone–binding globulin synthesis, therefore lowering total testosterone.[1] To put that simply, metabolic syndrome doesn't bode well for bedroom romance.

Liam wanted to deal with the condition naturally by changing his diet—he wasn't interested in lifelong prescriptions. He told me that he'd been eating the same kind of meals for the last few decades. When I asked him if he was open to making changes, he responded, "Sure, why not? I've been trying other things and not getting results." So we agreed to take baby steps, starting with returning to the grocery store. This time, I got to lead.

Liam and I mainly stuck to the perimeter of the store. We selected fresh fruits and dark, leafy green vegetables. We did buy some frozen vegetables for the sake of convenience, but we kept the packaged foods to a minimum. Instead, we purchased cold-water fish like wild-caught salmon, and we grabbed nuts and seeds for snacks. Liam was genuinely surprised at the importance of eating a variety of foods—he'd always thought the best way to lose weight was to stick with protein and avoid carbs.

After a few months, we agreed to assess his progress and condition to see if these diet and lifestyle adjustments benefited him. Although it was a challenge—especially when around his friends and work colleagues—he started seeing small changes that even his wife noticed. As a result, their next holiday card showed a much healthier version of Liam.

Liam had gathered his understanding about nutrition the way many of us do: by picking up info from friends, the gym, and social media. Unfortunately, Liam had gotten the idea that a healthy diet is packed with high protein and not much else—but actually, that misconception was causing considerable damage to his body. I've realized that many people are similar to Liam. They simply need better information about what it means to eat healthy. When you understand the nutrients your body requires to thrive and the foods that exhaust your body, you can eat your way to better health.

THE SAD DIET

Remember Bob Harper, the superstar personal trainer from *The Biggest Loser*? When I met him at a sporting event, I thought, "Wow, look how healthy and fit he is!" Then, only a few years later, I discovered he had a heart attack, which most would not have survived. I was initially surprised, but I was no longer shocked when I learned what he had been putting in his body—a high-protein, high-fat diet. Even though he did not eat the Standard American Diet (SAD), his diet had set him up for this event. Why? Most likely because it was *not well balanced* and made his cells angry.

Many of us grew up eating the Standard American Diet, also known as the Western diet. We were served it at school lunches, workplace cafeterias, and even in hospitals. It is characterized by a high intake of prepackaged meals, red meat, processed meats, fried foods, high-fat dairy products, refined grains, potatoes, and high-fructose corn syrup. Conversely, there is a low intake of fruits, vegetables, whole grains, nuts, and seeds.[2]

Most Westerners consume twenty-one meals every week, and if they follow the Standard American Diet, that means they consume pizza, burgers, burritos, takeout, and frozen foods on a regular basis. They're also consuming snacks like chips and ice cream. Three-fourths of Americans don't eat a single fruit on any given day, and nine out of ten don't reach the minimum recommended daily intake of vegetables.[3] The US Department of Agriculture estimates that 32 percent of our calories come from animal foods, 57 percent from processed plant foods, and only 11 percent from whole grains, beans, fruits, vegetables, and nuts.

That's the bad news. The good news is that it's relatively easy to make small, consistent changes in what you eat that will help optimize your wellbeing. But before we discuss specific foods to try, let's take a closer look at how your body interacts with the food you consume.

DIGESTION: HOW IT WORKS

So many aspects of our health and wellbeing can be traced back to the processes behind how we digest our food. One of my most common patient complaints is related to gut issues. When digestion works well, we absorb the nutrients from our food, excrete the waste, and our body manages to do it all without complaint. However, when something in this delicate process goes wrong, you can be sure you'll feel the effects.

THE DIGESTIVE TRACT

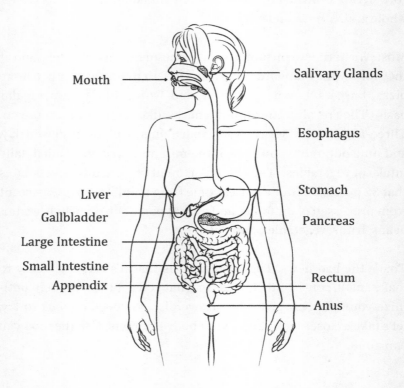

Mouth

Salivary Glands

Esophagus

Liver

Stomach

Gallbladder

Pancreas

Large Intestine

Small Intestine

Appendix

Rectum

Anus

Each part of the digestive system helps take food on a journey to be broken down into small pieces:

♦ As you chew, your **salivary glands** release enzymes that start breaking down your food.

♦ The food enters the **esophagus**; then *peristalsis* takes over, which means the muscle layer of the hollow organs automatically pushes the food and liquid through your gastrointestinal tract.

◆ As the esophageal sphincter relaxes, food is passed into the **stomach**. The stomach contains acids and enzymes to break down the food further.

◆ As food is passed from the stomach into the **small intestine**, the **pancreas** and **liver** help the intestine mix the food with digestive juices.

◆ Meanwhile, the **gallbladder** stores and releases bile made by your liver. Bile is responsible for digesting fats from your food.

◆ The small intestinal wall absorbs the digested nutrients into the **bloodstream**, and blood delivers these nutrients to the rest of the body.

◆ Undigested food and waste products are then pushed through the **large intestine**. The large intestine absorbs any remaining nutrients (with the help of our gut bacteria) and water while the remainder is pushed out of the body as stool.

It can take six to eight hours for food to pass through your stomach and small intestine. Further digestion, nutrient absorption, and waste elimination can take up to thirty-six hours. Depending upon the individual, the entire process could take up to five days. That means your Thanksgiving feast can stick with you for the better part of the following week!

But let's click that microscope lens up another notch and zoom in even closer. Within our digestive tract, there is an entire world made of trillions of microbes.

THE GUT MICROBIOME

The gut microbiome consists of a hundred trillion microbes colonizing your human gut wall lining. Yes, you read that right: a hundred *trillion*. This microbiome is affected by your diet, hygiene, geographic location, cultural practices, antibiotics, illness, stress, and overall lifestyle habits.[4] These microbes, or bacteria, comprise your gut flora, and they can be beneficial or harmful. Beneficial bacteria can help break down nutrients, make them usable for the body, stimulate your immune system, and help protect your cells.

On the other hand, harmful bacteria resulting from a poor diet, amongst other things, can adversely affect your body, triggering diseases such as irritable bowel disease, obesity, diabetes, carcinoma, arthritis, anxiety, and depression.[5] Although what you eat significantly affects your gut flora, it doesn't change overnight. So don't expect a single salad to crowd out the harmful bacteria if you regularly eat the SAD. Instead, consistently eating a whole, predominantly plant-based diet is the best way to repopulate your gut with the good guys. Several studies inform us that diet affects our microbiome and, ultimately, our body's ecosystem.[6]

Why You Should Love on Your GI Tract

The GI tract is essential for more reasons than just enabling us to process food. In fact, ancient whole-body systems such as Ayurveda believe poor gut health is the root cause behind many diseases. This is partly because your gut has its own enteric nervous system that operates independently of the brain and spinal cord. This system is composed of a network of small *ganglia* (nerve cells) that lie within the walls of your esophagus, stomach, and small and large intestines—in some ways making it your "second brain." However, the gut is responsible for so much more than simply digesting food and communicating with the brain.

The **gut acts as an intestinal barrier against pathogens**. Think of pathogens as bad guys: they're microorganisms and toxins that cause disease. So naturally, you don't want those pathogens to get into your bloodstream. But there's good news: you have *enterocytes*, intestinal cells which make up your gut lining to protect you from those nasty pathogens. When your gut lining is healthy, your enterocytes prevent pathogens from polluting your bloodstream.

But if your gut lining is damaged, some of those pathogens will invade from a "leaky gut." Those pathogens will then travel into other parts of your body, which can result in disease and impair your body's functions. Therefore, the *integrity of the gut lining is paramount.*

Now, it follows that if all sorts of harmful viruses and bacteria are getting into your bloodstream, you're going to get sick a lot. For that reason, the **gut plays a massive role in your immunity**. If your gut is full of beneficial bacteria, your immune system is likely to be strong. A weak gut lining, however, can contribute to many diseases, including autoimmune disorders.

Your gut bacteria also play an important role in **breaking down and metabolizing your food**. The bacteria take care of things the body can't do on its own, such as digesting fiber. Your body, surprisingly enough, doesn't have the enzymes needed to break down fiber; we have to rely on our gut bacteria to do that for us. Beneficial bacteria feed on fiber to produce something called *short-chain fatty acids* (SCFA), which, in turn, feed the colon's cells, reduce gut inflammation, and improve digestion. What does that mean in simple terms? It means a healthy bowel movement without a lot of gut discomfort.

Here's the point: without a healthy gut microbiome, *your body can't properly digest your food and utilize its nutrients.*

Healthy Food, Happy Gut

How exactly does the food we eat change our metabolism and our gut bacteria? To start with, a meat-heavy and saturated-fat diet isn't helping your #CellCare. Likewise, an animal-based diet can increase harmful bacteria, leading to chronic low-grade tissue inflammation.[7] (Remember, in Chapter Two, we discussed how inflammation could cause issues like joint pain, asthma, diabetes, cancer, and even mental health disorders.) However, a plant-based diet rich in grains, legumes, fruits, and vegetables promotes our gut bacteria's diverse and stable ecosystem.[8]

But it's not just your body that is impacted by the health of your gut; it's also your mind. **A healthy gut leads to a healthy brain**. There is a two-way communication channel between your gut and your brain via the vagus nerve. If you regularly experience "brain fog," memory loss, anxiety, or fatigue, there's a good chance your gut needs some attention. That's because your gut affects the production of serotonin, dopamine, and GABA (i.e., some of your "happy hormones") that influence both cognitive and emotional wellbeing.[9]

In other words, if you're continually eating processed food, your gut bacteria may negatively affect your mental headspace.

And since we're talking about the health of your gut, this is a good time to bring up the "Three Ps"—you've probably heard of one of them, but the other two deserve some attention as well.

Prebiotics, Probiotics, Postbiotics

The Three Ps—prebiotics, probiotics and postbiotics—are the trifecta for gut health and essential to the human body. They protect your gut from harmful bacteria, improve your digestion, and regulate your immune system. But what's the difference between them and where can you find them?

Prebiotics are the fiber that your good bacteria digests and uses as *fuel* for probiotics. They help increase the number and diversity of your microbiome and are found in foods such as apples, almonds, onions, leeks, bananas, legumes, and artichokes.

Probiotics (there's the well-known one) are your *working* beneficial bacteria that help aid digestion, prime your immune system, and reduce the growth of pathogenic organisms. Key sources include fermented foods such as kefir, kimchi, yogurt, and sauerkraut.

Postbiotics are the *metabolites* (beneficial chemicals) produced by your gut bacteria that play different roles in your health. For example, one type of postbiotic, SCFAs, maintain your gut lining, decrease inflammation, and send signals to your brain.

Given all the critical ways your GI tract affects your overall health, the gut has rightly become a significant focus of health and wellness in the past decade. Still, you don't necessarily need fancy or expensive products to improve your gut health. One of the best steps you can take for your GI tract is also one of the most straightforward: nourish it with whole foods.

NUTRITION FOR CELLULAR HEALTH

Some of the factors that impact your digestion and nutrient absorption are outside your control—but others *are* within your control. When you understand more about these nutrients, you'll have a much clearer sense of what foods will fuel your body.

WELLBEING FOOD PYRAMID

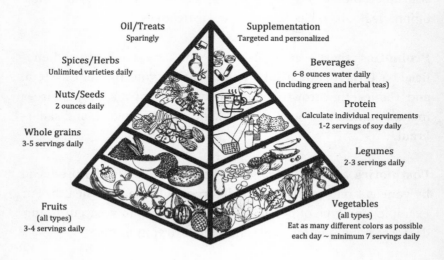

Oil/Treats
Sparingly

Supplementation
Targeted and personalized

Spices/Herbs
Unlimited varieties daily

Beverages
6-8 ounces water daily
(including green and herbal teas)

Nuts/Seeds
2 ounces daily

Protein
Calculate individual requirements
1-2 servings of soy daily

Whole grains
3-5 servings daily

Legumes
2-3 servings daily

Fruits
(all types)
3-4 servings daily

Vegetables
(all types)
Eat as many different colors as possible
each day ~ minimum 7 servings daily

Ideally, your nutrition will lean heavily on fruits and vegetables, which provide essential micronutrients, along with fiber. The next largest category would be whole grains and legumes, which provide important fiber and energy. Protein—rather than being your main source of calories—would fall in the middle; protein is an important source of amino acids. Toward the top of your nutritional intake pyramid, you would have your beverages and the spices you want to flavor the foods already mentioned. At the very top of that pyramid—like the star on a Christmas tree—you would enjoy treats in small amounts and supplement your nutrition with vitamins you're not otherwise able to get through your food.

Let's break down two of the more familiar nutritional categories: **macronutrients** and **micronutrients**.

- ◆ **Macronutrients** are the primary nutrients you need in large amounts to fuel and energize your body. You are probably familiar with these: carbohydrates, proteins, and fats.

- ◆ **Micronutrients** are the nutrients your body needs in smaller amounts to maintain tissue and cellular function and prevent disease. These include vitamins, minerals, and water.

Let's uncomplicate the macronutrients first.

Carbs Are Not the Enemy

Carbohydrates—composed of starch, sugar, and dietary fiber—are your body's primary fuel source and should consist of **45 to 65**

percent of your diet. They are found in vegetables, fruits, nuts, seeds, grains, and legumes. *Simple carbohydrates*—like fruit juice concentrate, high-fructose corn syrup, and some sugary cereals— are made of easy-to-digest sugars that are quickly absorbed through our gut and spike blood sugar levels. (That's not great.) On the other hand, *complex carbohydrates* are found in *whole grains, legumes, and vegetables*. These types of carbs are higher in fiber—which is highly beneficial to your body—and take longer to digest, so they don't spike your blood sugar.

The fiber from the complex carbs is an integral part of your diet because it benefits your gut bacteria and reduces your risk of chronic disease. Yet, less than 5 percent of people get the recommended amount of fiber. On average, intake should be 25 grams per day for women and 38 grams per day for men. A meat-heavy diet will often have no fiber; that was the case for Liam, which was one of the main reasons his body was functioning poorly. Of note: there is no fiber in meat, dairy, or sugar.

How do you know if you're not getting enough fiber? If you find yourself hungry after a meal, you might be lacking adequate fiber. This might also be the case if you're consistently bloated and constipated. Lack of fiber can affect cholesterol levels and contribute to high blood pressure; it can even hinder your attempts to lose weight.

Our beneficial bacteria love fiber, and they turn it into the SCFAs previously mentioned. Why should we want those SCFAs? Because SCFAs can:

♦ Increase fat burning and decrease fat storage.[10]

♦ Decrease cholesterol production and risk of heart disease.[11]

♦ Help with blood sugar control.[12]

♦ Have an anti-inflammatory effect and protect against
digestive disorders.[13]

SCFAs are found in *resistant starches* (whole-grain cereals, brown
rice, lentils, and beans), *pectin* (apples, carrots, and oranges), and
inulin (onions and asparagus). But nutrition is not just about the
fiber; a wellbeing lifestyle also prioritizes micronutrients.

#**CellCare:** Here are my top ten choices for low-carb,
high-fiber vegetables and fruits:

♦ **Bell peppers:** Contain antioxidants called carotenoids, high in vitamins A and C, protect against
oxidative damage, and reduce inflammation.[14]

♦ **Cauliflower:** Contains vitamins K and C and, like
other cruciferous vegetables, is associated with a
reduced risk of heart disease and cancer.[15]

♦ **Cucumbers:** Contain a compound called cucurbitacin E, which may protect against cancer and
support brain health.[16]

♦ **Brussels sprouts:** Contain vitamins K and C and
may reduce cancer risk.[17]

- **Radishes:** Contain vitamin C and may reduce the risk of breast cancer by modifying the way estrogen is metabolized.[18]

- **Onions:** Contain the antioxidant quercetin that lowers blood pressure and LDL cholesterol levels.[19]

- **Cabbage:** Contains vitamins C and K and may reduce the risk of esophageal and stomach cancer.[20]

- **Avocados:** Contain vitamin C, folate, and potassium; they also help you lose weight because they're a source of fiber, and the good fats they contain help reduce cardiovascular risks.[21]

- **Berries:** Source of antioxidants, potassium, vitamin C, and phytochemicals that can prevent chronic disease.

- **Honeydew:** High in vitamin C and potassium, which helps maintain good blood pressure and healthy metabolism.

When people think about avoiding carbs, they often don't understand the difference between good and bad carbs. White pasta, white rice, cereals, crackers, and white bread are all *refined* and have detrimental effects on your health. You might think they taste good, but they're not worth the trade-off when they lead to chronic inflammation, Type 2 diabetes, high blood pressure,[22] blood sugar spikes, acne,[23] allergies, mood swings,[24] difficulty concentrating,[25] bloating, and bone loss.[26]

#CellCare: Use the opportunity to incorporate fiber at every meal. For example, for breakfast, make a smoothie with avocados and spinach. At lunch, incorporate dark leafy greens and quinoa. For dinner, try working in some roasted veggies like carrots, broccoli, and Brussels sprouts. As you incorporate more vegetables into your meals, your body may need some time to adjust to the added fiber, so cooked vegetables will be easier on your digestive tract.

We often don't think about fruits and vegetables being a source of carbohydrates—typically, we think all of our carbs come from grains, and many people assume that all carbs are bad. That's not quite true. A "whole" grain is a grain that contains three components: bran, endosperm, and germ—and whole grains are good for you. All three components in whole grains contain many nutrients that are beneficial to our cells:

♦ **Bran:** The fiber-filled outer layer that contains B vitamins, iron, zinc, magnesium, antioxidants, and phytochemicals.

♦ **Germ:** The nutrient-packed core that contains vitamins B and E, healthy fats, antioxidants, and phytochemicals.

♦ **Endosperm:** The starchy middle layer that contains carbohydrates and a small amount of protein and vitamins.

However, when we process grains into their "white" versions (think: white rice, white flour, crackers, cookies, many cereals), we remove everything but the starchy endosperm, which causes loss of most of its nutrients.

WHOLE GRAIN VERSUS REFINED GRAIN

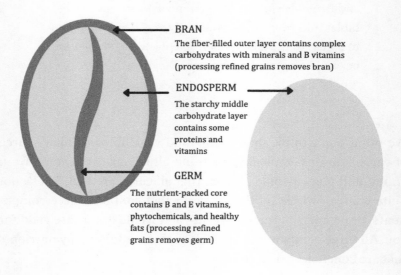

BRAN
The fiber-filled outer layer contains complex carbohydrates with minerals and B vitamins (processing refined grains removes bran)

ENDOSPERM
The starchy middle carbohydrate layer contains some proteins and vitamins

GERM
The nutrient-packed core contains B and E vitamins, phytochemicals, and healthy fats (processing refined grains removes germ)

A wellbeing lifestyle contains lots of whole grains. Skip the Wonder Bread and opt instead for multi-grain bread, lentils, or brown rice—all those delicious, high-fiber options that will make your microbiome happy.

#CellCare: Whole grains include oats, amaranth, buckwheat, barley, quinoa, brown or colored rice, sorghum, and rye. (Just to name a few!) An easy way to incorporate whole grains in your diet is batch cooking for the week, adding whole grains as a salad base, making a grain bowl, or switching out your cereal for some steel cut oats.

Many fad diets lead you to believe that carbs are the bad guy—the main culprit behind weight gain and inflammation. While that may be true for *processed* grains, whole grains have many health benefits, including fighting disease, lowering systemic inflammation,[27] reducing cardiovascular risk,[28] aiding weight loss, and decreasing the risk of mortality.[29] In addition, carbohydrates are an essential macronutrient for the body and important for well-balanced #CellCare. For this reason, substituting whole grains, vegetables, and fruits for refined carbohydrates is better for cellular health than a no-carb diet.

Make Unsaturated Fat Your New BFF

The next macronutrient you should include in your diet is fat. You need twice as many fats as you do protein! Fat is vital for many processes in the body, including absorbing vitamins and minerals and producing energy. Therefore, consider anywhere from **15 to 30 percent** good fat in your diet. However, not all fat is created equal. We want to *avoid* fats that make our cells angry, and seek out good fats that help our cells function optimally.

What are the bad fats? Overeating **saturated fat** can raise total cholesterol, LDL levels (which is bad cholesterol), and inflammation within the body,[30] increasing the risk for heart disease and Type 2 diabetes. Common sources of saturated fat include meat, chicken, pork, and dairy products.

There's another type of fat that is even worse than saturated fat: **trans fat.** Trans fat has no nutritional value, and in 2015, the US Food and Drug Administration stated that *artificial trans fat is not recognized as safe to eat.* It's often found in fried foods, processed snacks, and baked goods: for instance, frozen pizza dinners, breakfast doughnuts, and microwaved popcorn.

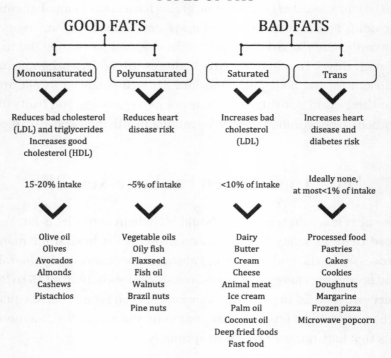

TYPES OF FAT

GOOD FATS		BAD FATS	
Monounsaturated	Polyunsaturated	Saturated	Trans
Reduces bad cholesterol (LDL) and triglycerides Increases good cholesterol (HDL)	Reduces heart disease risk	Increases bad cholesterol (LDL)	Increases heart disease and diabetes risk
15-20% intake	~5% of intake	<10% of intake	Ideally none, at most<1% of intake
Olive oil Olives Avocados Almonds Cashews Pistachios	Vegetable oils Oily fish Flaxseed Fish oil Walnuts Brazil nuts Pine nuts	Dairy Butter Cream Cheese Animal meat Ice cream Palm oil Coconut oil Deep fried foods Fast food	Processed food Pastries Cakes Cookies Doughnuts Margarine Frozen pizza Microwave popcorn

By contrast, consuming plant-based **monounsaturated fat (MUFA)** may help lower your risk of cardiovascular disease and mortality. Sources of MUFAs include olive oil, avocados, and most nuts and seeds.

Polyunsaturated fats (PUFA)—omega-3 and **omega-6**—are required for maintaining healthy cell structure and processes. Your body needs these essential fatty acids, and the only way to get them is through your food. Most of us are getting far too much omega-6 and hardly any omega-3. Ideally, we would consume omega-6 and omega-3 in a 4:1 ratio. Unfortunately, most American diets are 10:1 and sometimes even 30:1. So how do we correct that ratio?

To improve the ratio, increase omega-3 fatty acids by eating more foods like ground flax seeds, soybeans, walnuts, sunflower seeds, chia seeds, and hemp seeds. On the other hand, the single most important thing people can do to decrease their omega-6 fatty acids is avoid processed seed and vegetable oils—canola, soybean, safflower, or corn oil—often used in restaurant kitchens and processed foods.

> **#CellCare:** Avoid the *bad fats:* trans fats are the worst and saturated fats aren't far behind. Choose the *good fats:* monounsaturated fats and polyunsaturated fats are your friends!

Protein (You're Probably Overeating)

The epicenter of a typical American's plate is protein. We *love* protein in this country. Many foods are marketed primarily as a source of high protein. Additionally, many fad diets are incredibly heavy on protein consumption. But the truth is, our body does not require nearly as much protein as most of us think.

Protein requirements vary across your lifespan. As a guideline, the average adult should consume **0.8 grams of protein/kg of body weight** each day and protein should account for **15 percent of your overall daily food intake**. Let's take a day in the life of our friend Liam. For breakfast, he would have a pre-workout protein shake (30 grams of protein), post-workout protein shake (30 grams of protein), lunch with grilled chicken breast (54 grams of protein), and dinner composed of a burger (27 grams of protein) and another shake (30 grams of protein). In total, he had 171 grams of protein in a day, while his body only needed 70 grams. That is over double the amount! And he was not a professional athlete—he was a financial advisor trying to stay healthy.

Even if you aren't adding in extra protein shakes, look at the protein you consume at breakfast, lunch, and dinner. It may be above your requirement, especially if you are eating the Standard American Diet.

#CellCare: Calculate your average protein needs.

Weight in pounds divided by 2.2 = weight in kg

Weight in kg x 0.8 gram/kg = X grams of protein

Note: If you are an athlete, under stress, pregnant, or recovering from illness, these needs may increase, and therefore the 0.8 can be increased accordingly to between 1 and 1.8.

What exactly is wrong with excess protein consumption? High protein consumption is a concern because excess protein is not used efficiently by the body. As a result, extra protein burdens our organs, specifically our kidneys, liver, and bones. In addition, the body cannot store protein, so once your body's needs are met, any excess amino acids from protein are converted to carbohydrates or fat. All of that excessive protein may be the reason for your weight gain. In addition, high-protein, high-meat diets are associated with an increased risk of coronary heart disease and cancer.[31]

#CellCare: Integrating plant-based protein into your diet may be an effective way to reduce saturated fat that goes hand in hand with animal sources. These plant-based sources may include:

- **Tofu and edamame:** Contain between 10 to 19 grams of protein per 3.5 ounces and is a source of calcium and iron.

- **Lentils:** Contain 18 grams of protein per 1 cup and are rich in folate, manganese, iron, and antioxidants.

- **Beans:** Contain 15 grams of protein per 1 cooked cup and are rich in fiber, iron, folate, potassium, manganese, and phosphorus.

- **Nuts, seeds, and nut butter:** Contain approximately 6 grams of protein per serving and are sources of calcium, magnesium, and B vitamins.

- **Vegetables:** Contain approximately 5 grams of protein per 1 cooked cup (the highest amounts are in asparagus, sweet potatoes, Brussels sprouts, broccoli, and spinach) and are a source of phytonutrients—which we're about to discuss in detail!

Don't get too hung up on macronutrient percentages. They are just meant as a starting point. If your body feels gross after eating a greasy pizza, or if you feel energized and strong after a nutrient-dense salad, your body is giving you information about what it needs. Your cells will tell you what you need if you are willing to listen to them.

MICRONUTRIENTS

Okay—that covers our macronutrients. But what about the micronutrients you also need?

Micronutrients include about thirty vitamins and minerals that your body cannot produce on its own. As discussed in Chapter Three, our bodies need a range of minerals and vitamins for good cellular health. Most of these minerals and vitamins can be supplied through a well-balanced diet, complete with plenty of fruits, vegetables, whole grains, legumes, and healthy fats.

But let's take a closer look here at another essential micronutrient category: phytonutrients.

Phytonutrients

Phytonutrients are chemical compounds produced by plants. They're beneficial because they enhance our immunity and improve the communication between cells, a process we described in Chapter Two. Phytonutrients also repair DNA damage when we're exposed to toxins; you can think of them as microscopic EMTs in our bodies, rushing to the side of damaged DNA and bandaging them up to help them heal. As much as we'd like to avoid toxins entirely, we don't live in a bubble, so consuming phytonutrients is essential. They also reduce inflammation, which is a nasty byproduct of many of our lifestyle choices.

All in all, phytonutrients play a huge role in fighting disease and keeping your cells working properly.[32] Let's discuss key ones that you should know about.

ESSENTIAL PHYTONUTRIENTS AND THEIR FOOD SOURCES

Carotenoids are pigments found in fruits and vegetables that produce their bright orange, yellow, and red colors. They act as antioxidants to support our immune systems by combating harmful free radicals and tissue damage. The following is a list of carotenoids and their food sources:

ESSENTIAL PHYTONUTRIENTS: CAROTENOIDS

- ♦ β-**carotene** is a provitamin that can be converted to vitamin A. It may improve cognitive function,[33] skin health,[34] and eye health[35] and protect against certain cancers.[36] Sources include dark leafy greens, carrots, sweet potatoes, broccoli, cantaloupe, cilantro, parsley, paprika, and coriander.

♦ α-**carotene** also helps make vitamin A and is found in pumpkin, butternut squash, tangerines, napa cabbage, avocados, and bananas.

♦ **Lycopene** has been linked to a lower risk of prostate cancer and may lower your risk of heart disease[37] and stroke.[38] It can be found in tomatoes, watermelon, papaya, guava, and pink grapefruit.

♦ **Lutein and zeaxanthin** are antioxidants beneficial to eye[39] and skin[40] health. Key sources include parsley, spinach, broccoli, kiwis, grapes, peas, and kale.

All of the above foods are absorbed more effectively when eaten with healthy fats, like avocados, nuts, or olive oil.

#**CellCare:** Carotenoid-rich foods protect your eye health, helping you absorb blue light; promote cardiovascular health, preventing blood vessel blockages; support immune health, fighting off infections; and lower your risk of certain cancers.

Another category of phytonutrients is **flavonoids**, which are potent antioxidants found in a variety of plant foods, tea, and dark chocolate. A flavonoid-rich diet can help prevent chronic disease and increase longevity.[41]

ESSENTIAL PHYTONUTRIENTS: FLAVONOIDS

♦ **Flavones (luteolin, apigenin)** have anti-inflammatory and neuroprotective effects (i.e., they help prevent cognitive decline)[42] and are found in parsley, celery, and hot peppers.

♦ **Flavonones (hesperetin, eriodictyol, naringenin)** are found in citrus fruits and are associated with cardiovascular health, helping you manage weight and cholesterol.

♦ **Flavonols (quercetin, kaempferol)** are anti-inflammatory, improve exercise performance, and lower blood sugar. They are found in onions, leeks, berries, apples, and all teas.

♦ **Flavan-3-ols (catechins)** may help cardiovascular[43] and brain health[44] and are found in green, black, and white tea.

The simplest way to optimize the functioning of your cells with more flavonoids comes back to some advice you've already heard quite a few times: eat more fruits and vegetables. If you find these lists overwhelming or the information hard to remember, make that your single take away: lots of fruits and vegetables will check off most of your body's essential nutrient boxes. Bottom line, eat the rainbow. (Just not the Skittles kind!)

But that doesn't mean we're done with the lists. Finally, there are additional phytonutrients with their own special health benefits:

OTHER ESSENTIAL PHYTONUTRIENTS

- **Ellagic acid** is an antioxidant with anti-inflammatory properties that may help reduce cancer risk[45] and prevent brain disease, like Alzheimer's.[46] It's found in raspberries, strawberries, blackberries, grapes, pomegranates, walnuts, pistachios, and cashews.

- **Resveratrol** is excellent for cardiovascular and brain health due to its antioxidant and anti-inflammatory properties. It also has anti-tumor effects by inhibiting cancer cell growth and promoting cell death. It can be found in berries, grapes, pistachios, and peanuts.

- **Phytoestrogens and isoflavones (genistein, glycitein, daidzein)** help lower breast, endometrial, and prostate cancer risk. They may also help prevent heart disease and osteoporosis. They are found in soy products, legumes, and vegetables such as green peas, cabbage, and broccoli sprouts.

- **Glucosinolate (indole-3-carbinol)** may have antibacterial, antiviral, and antifungal properties, and it can lower your cancer risk.[47] It is found in cruciferous vegetables, including cabbage, kale, broccoli, and Brussels sprouts.

Your Best Source for Micronutrients

The best source of micronutrients—our vitamins, minerals, and phytonutrients—(once again) is a variety of fruits, vegetables, whole grains, nuts, and seeds. To get the most out of your produce, buy organic if it's within your budget. Nonorganic produce can contain toxins from pesticides, and they're often less nutrient-dense than organic produce.[48] If you're concerned about the cost of organic produce, check the frozen aisle. Frozen organic fruits and vegetables are often cheaper than fresh organic produce.

#CellCare: Each year, the Environmental Working Group releases a resource called "Dirty Dozen; Clean Fifteen" which lists foods that contain the highest residual amounts of pesticides. From this list you can determine what foods are okay to buy non organic. It can be hard to remember that list when you're away from the website, so I recommend taking a screenshot and referencing it while you're shopping for produce.

If you're not used to eating many fruits and vegetables, get excited: there are so many delicious ways to prepare these foods that will satisfy your palate and make your body feel nourished. Also, remember that you can use as many spices as you want to flavor your food.

Here's the bottom line: eating nutritionally dense, real food will support your cells, and ultimately your body, in functioning properly. A body that doesn't get what it needs won't feel full or satisfied, and it clamors for more. In contrast, when your body receives the nutrients it needs, it will feel satisfied after eating.

FOOD VILLAINS AND FAD DIETS

How did we go so wrong? As a society, why do we consume so many junk foods and nutrient-deficient meals when there are so many healthy foods to eat?

For one, the Industrial Revolution made processed foods a fixture in the American landscape. The food industry developed ways to preserve and process foods for a longer shelf-life, but unfortunately, many of the added ingredients were also extremely addictive, such as trans fats and high-fructose corn syrup. The combination of sugar and fat in highly processed foods activates a part of the brain associated with compulsive behavior.[49] It goes a little like this: when you eat your favorite processed food, your brain gives you a hit of dopamine—a high. This creates an associated pleasure with consuming the food. However, that small dopamine hit with just one cookie is not enough over time, so you start to eat more and more cookies. Ultimately, that initial high creates a slump as your gut struggles to metabolize the processed food, even while your body continues to crave needed nutrients. At this point, the dopamine effect in your brain makes it difficult to resist the urge, making it very challenging to give up the craving. Big food industries know the addictive nature of processed food, and they capitalize on it.

Some of the most tempting foods aren't doing you any good when it comes to your #CellCare. So, as you move your culinary nourishment in a healthier direction, watch out for these food villains who want to lure you to the dark side.

Sugar Is Not Sexy

Your dentist was onto something when he told you to limit your sugar intake. It tastes good going down, but the subsequent inflammation wreaks havoc on your cells. Not only does it negatively impact dental health, but it can also accelerate cognitive decline,[50] cellular aging,[51] and increase the risk of depression,[52] cancer,[53] and heart disease.[54]

Believe it or not, there are *over fifty* different names for sugar. You can't possibly memorize all those names (or maybe you can) but do your best to avoid processed and artificial sweeteners, such as sucrose, cane sugar or cane syrup, corn syrup, fructose, and/or aspartame. Whenever possible, use natural forms of sugar, such as dates, maple syrup, or honey, to satisfy your sweet tooth.

Food Additives

Food additives are used to preserve and enhance the flavor and texture of food. However, they do come with adverse effects. They alter our gut microbiome, cause allergic reactions, affect immune health, and contribute to chronic disease.

When picking up food at the grocery store, don't forget to read the labels and watch out for these nasty additives:

FOOD ADDITIVES TO AVOID

♦ Monosodium glutamate (MSG)

♦ Artificial food coloring (Blue 1, Yellow 5, Red 40)

♦ Sodium nitrite

♦ Guar gum

- Carrageenan

- High-fructose corn syrup

- Artificial sweeteners

- Sodium benzoate

- Xanthan gum

Many of us have no idea that some of the unpleasant symptoms we're experiencing are from these additives. For instance, guar gum—found in salad dressings, soups, and yogurt—is okay in small amounts, but if you have any gut health issues, you should avoid it, as it can cause gas, bloating, and cramps.[55] Additionally, carrageenan— which is found in ice cream, almond milk, and coffee creamers—may trigger inflammation and negatively impact digestive health.[56] The flavor enhancer MSG, found in Chinese food, cheese, canned soups, and fast foods like Chick-Fil-a and KFC, has been linked to obesity, liver damage, heart disease, nerve damage, and inflammation.[57]

Furthermore, even though the FDA considers xanthan gum safe for food consumption, it can't be digested by the body. You can find it in salad dressings, ice creams, and low-fat foods; plus, you may find it in toothpaste, shampoo, and even wallpaper glue and toilet bowel cleaners. I would be wary of it if you have digestive issues. Artificial food coloring is another additive found in cereals and candy; it's linked to behavioral changes including irritability, depression, and ADHD.[58]

Remember: take a look at what you are consuming *most* of the time, not some of the time, as your regular diet will have the greatest impact on your wellbeing.

How can you steer clear of food additives? Choosing whole foods and limiting packaged foods will benefit you by eliminating artificial ingredients such as preservatives and food coloring.

Milk Does Not Do a Body Good

Another food villain is one that's been paraded as a food hero for years. Bad news: dairy, a staple in the SAD, is not as good for us as we previously thought. In an extensive study, adults who consumed the most dairy were at a higher risk of total cardiovascular and cancer mortality.[59] When dairy was replaced with beans, whole grains, and nuts, the risk decreased. In addition, dairy has been linked to Parkinson's disease[60] and prostate cancer.[61] Yet another study determined that women who consumed a fourth to a third of a cup of cow's milk per day had a 30 percent increased chance of breast cancer.[62] And (I'm sorry, cheese lovers!) another study found that a diet containing high consumption of American cheddar and cream cheese resulted in a 53 percent higher risk for breast cancer.[63] (For those who don't know, one in eight women develop breast cancer; the youngest I've diagnosed is an eighteen-year-old with no inborn genetic mutations.)

Even dairy products that seem healthy (thanks to good marketing), such as Greek yogurt with live cultures, aren't good for you. Furthermore, we've learned that dairy products have little to no benefit for bones.[64] All those "Got Milk?" ads are great marketing but don't convey the whole nutritional truth.

Okay, that's the bad news. But there's good news: there are plenty of other great sources for calcium intake. Plant-based foods, fortified cereals and bread, kale, and broccoli are all excellent natural sources rich in calcium and don't come with chronic illnesses in tow. To reap the full benefits of calcium you also require an adequate intake of vitamin D, vitamin K, and magnesium.

#CellCare: Here are some top calcium-rich foods—that *aren't* dairy:

♦ Chia seeds

♦ Sesame seed

♦ Beans

♦ Lentils

♦ Almonds

♦ Leafy greens, like kale and collard greens

♦ Edamame

♦ Tofu

♦ Figs

Advanced Glycation End Products

You might have noticed that I promote an exclusively plant-based diet—and there's a reason for that. One of the food villains that you should be aware of is advanced glycation end products (AGEs), otherwise known as glycotoxins. When consumed, they increase inflammation and oxidative stress, contributing to degenerative diseases.[65] The acronym is appropriate since they tend to cause signs of premature aging and—bad news for steak lovers—AGEs are ingested via meats cooked at high temperatures, dairy products, and foods with a high sugar content. Uncooked animal-derived foods naturally contain AGEs, and cooking—especially grilling, broiling, roasting, and frying—promotes the formation of new AGEs. Bacon and parmesan cheese are two extremely high sources. In the end, AGEs make your cells become stiffer and dysfunctional as the proteins are negatively impacted and your extracellular matrix is damaged.

Fad Diets

After learning about the SAD and the negative consequences of sugar, dairy, food additives, and AGEs, you might be considering changing your diet. But what kind of diet should you choose? First, let me give you a piece of advice: avoid fad diets. Some people go on them to feel better, but most people go on them to *look* better. Fad diets promise quick results but do not educate consumers about the lifestyle needed for sustained health benefits. Furthermore, fad diets promise exaggerated results, such as rapid weight loss or detoxification.[66] Although fad diets may improve your short-term results, they can lead to a nutritional imbalance that undermines your overall health.

The ketogenic diet (keto for short) is just one example of a fad diet that promises great things but significantly stresses your body. The keto diet is a high-fat, low-carb diet that promises rapid weight loss. This diet was initially developed to ease uncontrolled epileptic seizures—its high-fat content was thought to help reduce seizure activity in the brain. But this diet also has detrimental factors—it can cause constipation and headaches, increase the risk of heart disease, and eliminate many healthy foods from your everyday diet.[67]

Maybe these warnings about food villains and fad diets seem exaggerated. Perhaps you grew up eating junk food, dairy, and processed food—all of the worst culprits of the SAD—and you don't have a chronic disease yet. So, all in all, you might feel pretty fit. But, unfortunately, these nutritional choices do catch up with you. You are what you eat, and over time, your body becomes less able to handle unhealthy foods. I don't say that to be a killjoy, but as someone who has witnessed the consequences of poor diets on hundreds of thousands of damaged human cells.

The more sustainable approach to your diet is to simply practice eating real, whole foods consistently rather than trying fad diets. Focus on filling your plate with a colorful variety of fruits and vegetables, whole grains, and good fats. When you begin to nourish your body with real nutrients, you no longer have to count calories and you start craving good food.

What are practical ways to do this? Let's consider rituals that can help your culinary nourishment.

RITUALS FOR WELLBEING

Remember: rituals are small lifestyle tweaks that can create big results. Intentional changes to your culinary nourishment can literally transform (and even save!) your life. Let's consider how you can optimize your eating experience for more excellent health and wellbeing.

Mindfulness While Eating

Distracted eating can have negative consequences. Whether we eat on the go, mindlessly munch on snacks while watching a show, or shove in food during the middle of a stressful workday, most of us don't engage in mindful eating. As a result, we often eat more than we need or consume foods that offer us no real nutritional value.

By practicing *mindful* eating, you can make a healthy shift away from mindless eating. Eating mindfully not only helps you become healthier but also improves your enjoyment of food.

Try building more awareness of your sensory experiences during mealtime. For instance, science informs us that our sense of smell can stimulate activity in our GI tract, which will increase our nutrient uptake and improve digestion.[68] A study from France looked at the mindfulness eating habits of over 60,000 people and found that individuals with a propensity toward mindfulness were less likely to be obese or overweight.[69] You can incorporate mindfulness into your culinary nourishment by:

149

◆ Being mentally present during the entire process of the meal, from preparation to cooking to indulging.

◆ Turning off all distractions—put away the cell phone and turn off the TV while you're eating.

◆ Taking three deep breaths before starting your meal to be fully present while eating.

◆ Inhaling the aroma of the food, chewing, and savoring the taste of each bite.

◆ Expressing gratitude both before and after your meal. Many people take a moment to give thanks before a meal, but we rarely think to do it afterward. Taking a "gratitude pause" after your meal can help you register the satisfaction you've gotten from it and help prevent you from additional snacking later.

Think of incorporating these mindfulness practices into the very substance of your meal. You can think of this as serving up a Wellbeing Lifestyle Plate: full of nutritious foods and characterized by its mindful eating rituals.

What might that look like?

◆ Around half of your plate—for breakfast, lunch, and dinner—will be fruits and vegetables, with a heavier emphasis on vegetables.

◆ Around a quarter of your plate will be whole grains (unprocessed and unrefined).

♦ Another quarter will be high-quality fats and protein.

♦ The goal is to get at least 10 servings of vegetables and fruits in your body per day. (Most people just get 2—and one of those is typically potatoes.)

♦ Try to get 5 to 7 servings of omega-3 fatty acids per day (olive oil, avocado, nut seeds, etc.).

WELLBEING LIFESTYLE PLATE

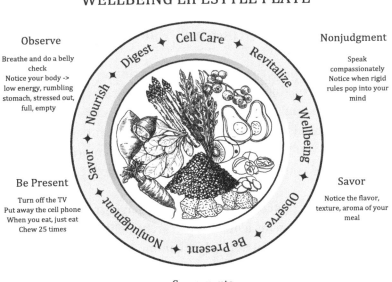

Observe
Breathe and do a belly check
Notice your body ->
low energy, rumbling stomach, stressed out, full, empty

Nonjudgment
Speak compassionately
Notice when rigid rules pop into your mind

Be Present
Turn off the TV
Put away the cell phone
When you eat, just eat
Chew 25 times

Savor
Notice the flavor, texture, aroma of your meal

Components
50% of colorful plate: vegetables > fruit
Whole grains = quinoa, amaranth, brown rice
Plant based protein = beans, lentils, soy
Avocados, olive oil, nuts/seeds
Herbs/spices

Ultimately, you're looking to create a predominately whole-food, plant-forward plate. If you choose to consume animal products, consider that more of a side than the centerpiece of your meal. You can find plant-forward recipes on my website, DrBhanote.com. Lastly, everything on your plate will be consumed with a mindful approach.

A Wellbeing Lifestyle Plate will not only help you fight cellular damage with its abundance of antioxidants, phytonutrients, vitamins, and minerals—it will also make your entire body run efficiently, thanks to its mindful eating approach.

Mise-en-place

Mise-en-place is a term used by chefs meaning "everything in its place." When cooking, the chef sets everything up at their workstation before cooking a meal. They have their vegetables, spices, oils, and everything else laid out before beginning the process of cooking. Give it a try: you'll find the experience becomes more efficient and enjoyable, and you might also feel like your favorite celebrity chef!

When you apply this concept to nutrition—laying out all your ingredients before preparing a meal—you can be deliberate about eating an entire rainbow of nutrients. It is common for people to consume the same breakfasts, lunches, and dinners on a weekly basis, meaning they may not be consuming a variety of phytonutrients, vitamins, and minerals. By practicing the ritual of mise-en-place, you will see the colors of your foods when they're laid out in front of you. At that point, it becomes easy to assess whether or not you have variety while planning or creating meals and be more thoughtful in your food preparation.

Food Selection and Food Labels

Start building awareness about the foods in your cart as you grocery shop. If you like the idea of eating your way toward greater wellbeing, try to select foods that do not come in packaging. However, if it does come in a box, look for minimally processed food, ideally with five ingredients or less. This will require you to read the nutrition label. Here are some things to look out for:

♦ If a food says fat-free, low-fat, sugar-free, or light, you can bet there's another ingredient in there to make it taste good—but that won't make your cells feel good.

♦ Always check serving size, servings per package, and calories.

♦ Read the entire nutrition facts label—you will see all the macronutrients we've talked about listed there.

♦ Limit the amount of sugar, sodium, and saturated and trans fats.

♦ Go for foods that are high in dietary fiber, calcium, iron, potassium, and vitamin D.

♦ Check that whole grains are actually whole grains. Look for the "whole grain stamp" from the Whole Grain Council, which affirms that the product will provide at least one serving of whole grains. If you see words like "wheat, semolina, multi-grain, durum wheat, organic flour, or stone ground," note that those are *packaging descriptions*, but the ingredients may be missing the benefits of the whole grain. The descriptions "enriched flour, wheat flour, cornmeal, bran, and wheat germ" are also deceptive: according to the Whole Grain Council, these words *never* describe whole grains.

♦ Check for all the different types of sugar—and try to limit to single-ingredient sugar and/or natural forms of sugar, like honey.

♦ Pay attention to notices like "non-GMO," which means *non*-genetically modified. (This is a good thing!)

> **#CellCare:** GMOs are living organisms which have been artificially manipulated through genetic engineering in a laboratory. This is generally done to increase food supply, create a longer shelf life, and make production cheaper, but they're essentially "franken-foods." The resulting genes—whether they are plant, animal, bacteria, or virus genes—do not occur in nature. GMOs are found in many processed foods that contain corn starch, corn syrup, corn oil, soybean oil, canola oil, and granulated sugar—to name a few. The results of most studies on GMO foods indicate that they may cause some toxic effects on your organs (liver, pancreas, kidneys, or reproductive organs). They also may alter your blood, immune, and biochemical pathways. Translation: the less of them you eat, the better!

Meal Planning and Food Prep

Many people simply feel too maxed out to do meal planning or food prep. It feels easier to grab takeout on the way home from work or a quick meal from the freezer. However, these habits can set you up to consume foods that cause more harm than good to your body. By planning your meals ahead of time, you can be deliberate about choosing foods and ingredients that you know will be good for you. Although this might take some time upfront, it can easily save you time later in your week because you won't be scrambling for ingredients or a dinner plan.

Food prep goes hand-in-hand with meal planning because it saves you time and money. It also keeps you from constantly eating out and eating unhealthy meals. You can devote a couple of hours to your meal planning and food prep on the weekend or any other time that works for you. Keep the following tips in mind to optimize your #CellCare:

◆ Incorporate a variety of colors and textures.

◆ Vary the different tastes (in Ayurveda, we identify sweet, sour, salty, spicy, bitter, and astringent, where each flavor provides a different benefit to the body and role in digestion).

◆ Stock your pantry with whole grains, legumes, and nut butters.

◆ Have a collection of spices and herbs for flavoring.

♦ Designate a space for recipes, like a notebook or digital recipes folder, so it's quick and easy to find recipes and meal plan.

Intermittent Fasting

One of the world's most popular health trends is intermittent fasting (IF), but does it actually improve your wellbeing? Studies indicate that IF can have powerful effects on your body, possibly extending your life. The IF style of eating does not dictate specific foods to be consumed, but it promotes a cycle of eating and fasting between meals. A common method is the 16/8, in which you fast for sixteen hours and then eat within an eight-hour window. Even so, you should consume nutrient-dense foods that can nourish your body's cells (as mentioned in the substances for good cellular health).

What is the impact of IF on your cells? The body undergoes several changes at the molecular and cellular level when it fasts. The first is *autophagy*, where your body initiates cellular repair by digesting and removing old and dysfunctional proteins that build up inside the cells.[70] IF also affects the function of your genes related to longevity and protects you against diseases of aging.[71] As you age, your body is exposed to more oxidative stress, resulting in unstable free radicals, which cause inflammation and many of the diseases we see commonly. Some studies have shown that IF can reduce oxidative stress and overall inflammation in your body.[72] Fasting also allows your body to increase growth hormone levels to benefit fat loss and muscle gain.[73]

These are just a few of the benefits of IF, and the list continues to grow. For example, one of the fascinating studies I have seen demonstrates that IF may increase levels of a brain hormone called BDNF (brain-derived neurotrophic factor), which can help counteract depression and improve cognitive function.[74]

The use of intermittent fasting is not recommended while pregnant or if you suffer from an eating disorder or diabetes. But, apart from that, IF has many benefits for your body and cellular health, making it a practice worth trying.

Ritucharya (Eat Seasonally)

Maybe you're accustomed to eating the same foods throughout the year, but if you want to optimize #CellCare, consider eating seasonally. In Ayurveda, Ritucharya loosely translates into seasonal guidelines. Using these ancient practices, we are guided that each season can have an effect on our bodies. In the winter, when you are bundled up with hats and gloves, eating an ice cream may not be pleasant—however, enjoying it in the summer can be a delicious way to cool your body off. Similarly, when you're lying out by the pool in the summer, who would want a hot bowl of ten bean soup? In the winter, on the other hand, a warm stew can give your body needed nutrients and warmth.

Seasonal foods are often picked at peak freshness and can have more antioxidants and vitamins compared to out-of-season food. They also just taste better! Nature has its own way of helping us eat healthy by giving us different foods in different seasons. When we follow the seasons of nature, our body receives what it needs most. We hydrate our cells by eating water-rich foods like watermelon and cucumber in the summer. During the winter months, citrus gives us a boost in immunity as we battle cold and flu season. The winter also brings us an abundance of root vegetables and squashes, which are high in phytonutrients and warm our bodies. The health benefits of leafy greens can be reaped all year round. In the long run, eating within season can cause you to be healthier and prevent disease.

Spice Up Your Life

Spices are an excellent source of antioxidants due their high phenolic compounds. As well as enhancing your food's flavor and aroma, they can protect you from chronic illnesses. There is growing evidence that spices and herbs possess a variety of antioxidant, anti-inflammatory, antitumorigenic, anti-carcinogenic, and glucose- and cholesterol-lowering properties, as well as properties that affect cognition and mood. Researchers have found that including spices in your diet can help you live longer and decrease your risk of dying from cancer, ischemic heart disease and respiratory diseases.[75] Regularly consume spices and herbs like cinnamon, ginger, black pepper, turmeric, fenugreek, rosemary, garlic, cilantro, and parsley to boost your nutrition.

Eat Dark Chocolate!

Lest you think healthy eating is only about dark, leafy greens and high-fiber whole grains, let me enumerate the health benefits of dark chocolate.

Cacao, the main ingredient in chocolate, causes the brain to release multiple feel-good neurotransmitters, such as endorphins, dopamine, serotonin, and oxytocin. Not only is it good for your mood, but chocolate is also good for your brain: studies show dark chocolate can decrease neuroinflammation,[76] reduce stress while enhancing cognition and memory,[77] and increase neuroplasticity. It's even good for your gut, acting as a prebiotic that supports the growth of good bacteria in your GI tract.

The good news doesn't stop there. Cacao has multiple other beneficial ingredients that serve your body:

- *Theobromine* gives you an energy boost, can help reduce inflammation, and can lower blood pressure.[78]

- *Flavonoids* act as antioxidants: the darker the chocolate, the more antioxidants. This antioxidant effect can reduce inflammation and help your skin look more youthful and healthy.

- *Magnesium* is a cofactor in protein synthesis, muscle relaxation, and energy production.

- *Manganese, copper,* and *iron* are also minerals in chocolate that have beneficial effects.

These benefits largely come from dark chocolate—less so from milk chocolate. Pure cacao has a bitter taste, so chocolate makers usually use sugar and milk to balance the bitterness. Although milk chocolate is tasty, it has a reduced amount of cacao, which is replaced with ingredients that are not the best for your health. Dark chocolate, on the other hand, has a high percentage of cacao and lower amounts of sugar and milk.

So, to get a boost for your mood, increase your focus, help your body, and enhance your youthful appearance, opt for a single piece of *dark* chocolate. Enjoy the treat as you transition from a stressful workday into a relaxing evening. Savor the taste—and all its good effects!

Prepare Your Kitchen for Success

The kitchen can be an overwhelming place for some people. You buy groceries, only to have them go rotten before you finish eating them. You know you have an ingredient somewhere, but you can't find where it's stored. Organizing your refrigerator and pantry can save you time and money—not to mention, spare you some stress!

There's no right or wrong way to organize your refrigerator. However, you need a system that works for you, so consider making sure all the fresh fruits and vegetables are at eye level.

Invest in appropriate storage containers made from glass or stainless steel. These are not only eco-friendly but will also decrease your toxic burden and give you a place to organize your meal prep.

TRUE NOURISHMENT

Remember: when you understand the nutrients your body needs to thrive and are aware of foods that tax your body, you can eat your way to better health. A massive piece of the puzzle comes together simply by building more awareness—understanding how your body processes food, what it needs to thrive, what ingredients will best serve you, and being mindful when eating.

Food can be one of the most rewarding, satisfying, and socially rich experiences in our lives. It should be! When you incorporate more intention into your eating routines, you don't just set yourself up for better health—you set yourself up for greater wellbeing and satisfaction in one of life's most frequent experiences.

Reflect on Your #CellCare

Using these guiding questions, take a moment to build self-awareness and reflect on culinary nourishment in your life:

- ◆ Does your food selection reflect your attempts to eat healthy or your desire to eat for enjoyment? Do you believe you can do both at the same time?

- ◆ Do you often try new fad diets?

- ◆ Do you consume any products that negatively affect the health of your cells?

- ◆ Are you mindful when preparing and consuming your meals?

- ◆ Do you take the time to meal plan and eat seasonally?

- ◆ Have you organized your kitchen for true nourishment?

DESIGN YOUR WELLBEING

In the space below, note your thoughts about your culinary nourishment. What are some of your favorite foods? Do you eat a variety of foods? Are you getting adequate nutrients for cellular health? First, observe your current consumption, then consider rituals to incorporate culinary nourishment into your wellbeing. Then write down a ritual you want to incorporate into your life.

5

THE ART
OF MOVEMENT

"For me, exercise is more than just physical—it's thera-peutic."

~ MICHELLE OBAMA, ATTORNEY, AUTHOR, AND FOUNDER OF THE
"LET'S MOVE" PROGRAM TO ADDRESS CHILDHOOD OBESITY

WHEN I FIRST MET PEGGY, I WAS INSPIRED BY HER SENSE OF purpose. Peggy was a school social worker and dedicated her career to handling all sorts of situations involving children and families. She was always on the go but didn't move much outside of going from place to place for work. She usually ate her meals during staff meetings or while driving her car. Even though she ate plenty of fruits and vegetables, she still struggled with her energy, mood, and weight. After experiencing some additional symptoms that she suspected might be related to her weight, Peggy finally decided to seek me out.

Peggy explained to me that she felt depleted by the time she arrived home. "I know I should move my body more," she acknowledged, "but I haven't done anything to incorporate movement into my daily routine." Together, we examined some areas where she could add movement into her day.

When I asked Peggy to describe her typical twenty-four-hour day, I was struck by one of her habits in particular. Every day, while commuting home from work, Peggy talked to her best friend on the phone. Although her drive was only thirty minutes, she often spent closer to ninety minutes on the phone. Even after Peggy got home, she sat on the couch and continued the phone chat.

"Can we make better use of that extra call time?" I asked. "Is there any place on your commute home where you could stop the car and walk while talking, like a park or a trail?" She said there happened to be a new pedestrian bridge in her area, connected to some walking trails. So, rather than driving straight home after work, I suggested she consider stopping to walk this trail.

Initially, Peggy was reluctant to try the idea. She was accustomed to lounging around the house until dinnertime. I asked her if that was because her body felt truly physically exhausted.

"No, I'm not physically tired," she admitted. She described the various stresses of her workday and said the fatigue was probably mental and emotional. Finally, she said, "Honestly, I think I sit around because it's what I'm used to. It's a habit." She paused. "Maybe I could try to walk after all."

Walking is something almost everyone can do, but Peggy, like many people, had an all-or-nothing mentality about exercise. She believed she had to go to Orangetheory or do HIIT classes for adequate movement. However, walking didn't require her to go to the gym, purchase equipment, or even change her outfit. All she had to do was put on sneakers and go. Initially, the relative ease of walking made her think that it wasn't "real" exercise. But when I pointed out that *easy* is a great place to start if you're used to doing nothing, Peggy could see the potential benefits. The convenience factor began to appeal to her, and she became excited to get started.

Peggy also liked that she could walk without giving up the time she spent talking with her best friend. Instead, she attended to that meaningful relationship while taking care of herself. Making this new ritual felt well balanced.

Peggy and I discovered another great purpose to fuel her motivation: she told me that her biggest bucket list item was to take her grandchildren to Disneyland, but she'd almost given up on the idea. She was afraid that she wouldn't have the stamina to walk through the park several days in a row. However, the daily walking habit made her feel like she was making consistent progress toward getting stronger. She kept her goal constantly in mind: she wanted to be strong enough to do what she wanted to do—especially that Disneyland trip.

Like Peggy, most people know that the body needs movement to thrive, but often we don't realize how much flexibility we have with when, how, where, and what type of movement we can do. Of course you should exercise, but your movement rituals should also be sustainable and tailored to your lifestyle.

TOP 10 REASONS
WHY YOU SHOULD
BE PHYSICALLY ACTIVE

We know exercise is good for us and we'll be better for it—but many people don't know just *how* good exercise is for our bodies. So here are the top ten reasons why you should be physically active.

1. Boost Cardiovascular Endurance

Peggy wanted to increase her energy and stamina for that Disneyland trip. That's precisely what aerobic movement, or endurance exercises, will do for you. Endurance activities increase your breathing and heart rate. This type of movement not only improves your fitness and helps you accomplish daily tasks but can also delay or prevent many diseases that are common in older adults, such as diabetes, colon and breast cancers, heart disease, and others. Aerobic activities also play a vital part in the health of your heart, lungs, and circulatory system.

The only way for your muscles and organs to receive oxygen and nutrients is through blood circulation, and the best way to increase circulation is through movement. The heart must be trained like any other muscle, and movement provides this training through building cardiovascular endurance. This makes the heart pump blood efficiently, thus more effectively delivering nutrients throughout the body. With a strong and healthy heart, each heartbeat pushes out more blood and allows your body to best use your nutrients.

2. Feel More Energized

Ever notice that a lazy Saturday morning makes you feel sluggish for the entire day? That's because you haven't gotten your blood flowing. On the other hand, movement makes you feel energized both during exercise and afterward. Several things happen in your body during exercise to produce this boost in energy. First and foremost, your blood supply receives more oxygen when you get your heart pumping. This oxygenated blood continues to flow throughout the body for the rest of the day, allowing your body to function better and use energy more efficiently.

Exercise also fuels your mitochondria. In Chapter Three, we compared mitochondria—those little powerhouse organelles—to an iPhone battery. Your mitochondria create fuel from the food you eat and use oxygen from the air you breathe. Exercise stimulates your body to produce more mitochondria in your muscle cells, and more mitochondria means more energy.

Exercise also gives us a boost of hormones that makes us feel more energized. These hormones, called endorphins, also help relieve stress and pain—which contributes to that energy boost as well!

3. Get Better Sleep

Did you know that regular physical activity improves your sleep? You can quickly see improvements in your sleep with just thirty minutes of moderate aerobic exercise per day. That's because exercise increases quality of sleep and helps you fall asleep faster. Exercise also increases the time you spend in slow-wave sleep (a.k.a. deep sleep), which is the most restorative sleep.[1] It may also decrease daytime sleepiness because of the energy boost it stimulates throughout the day.

Why should exercise help you sleep better? Exercise increases your *sleep drive*, which is your desire to go to sleep. That's because your body wants to recuperate: your muscles need to repair themselves after being worked more than usual. It's also common to experience a drop in body temperature after a workout, which signals your body's sleep–wake cycle, cuing your body to fall asleep.

Additionally, people with sleeping troubles at night often find they are able to "turn their brains off" more quickly after exercise, since exercise releases muscle tension, decreases stress, and has been shown to have a positive effect on mood.

Keep this caveat in mind, though: exercise also produces endorphins that are energizing—so don't give yourself a cardio workout shortly before bed.

4. Increase Muscle Mass

Aerobic movement increases the amount of muscle tissue you have and is a countermeasure for muscle loss due to aging. That's helpful for more reasons than just sporting a six-pack. The more fat you have, the more inflammatory chemicals you produce. Regular exercise increases muscle mass and decreases fat mass (a.k.a. adipose cells), thus reducing chronic inflammation and cell damage.[2] At the same time, more muscle will increase blood flow and nutrient delivery and boost your energy, thanks to mitochondrial proliferation.[3]

5. Prevent Chronic Disease

People who don't move their bodies are at higher risk of developing chronic diseases. What kind of diseases? Lots of them: hypertension, type 2 diabetes, high cholesterol, obesity, coronary heart disease, along with increased risk of colon, breast, and possibly endometrial, lung, and pancreatic cancer. Even if you have no other risk factors or genetic disposition for these diseases, being physically inactive increases your risk, and that's backed up with three millennia of evidence.[4]

On the other hand, when you move your body, you increase the functional capacity of your cells. Also, you give your white blood cells a boost. White blood cells fend off disease, and the improved circulation that results from exercise allows white blood cells to circulate to areas that need immunity and healing.

6. Burn More Calories at Rest

Many of us exercise to burn calories, but there's a gift that keeps on giving when we work out: the *afterburn effect*. Technically, the afterburn effect is called EPOC (excess post-exercise oxygen consumption).[5] Basically, this means you continue to burn calories even after your workout has ended. How does that work?

After a workout, your body continues to remove lactic acid, repair muscles, and replenish ATP (energy made from your mitochondria). All of this post-workout activity means that you continue to burn calories and run a higher metabolism as your body repairs itself. Extra oxygen is also needed so the body can cool down, repair itself, and return to its resting state.

The most effective exercises for this afterburn effect are ones that use the whole body with dynamic moves—think squats, jumps, and burpees. This afterburn can last up to seventy-two hours, depending on the person and the workout. That means this incredible afterburn effect can keep you burning calories up to *three days* post-workout!

7. Improve Mental Focus

Exercise increases blood flow to the brain and is one of the easiest and most effective ways to improve concentration, motivation, and memory. Physical activity immediately boosts the brain's dopamine, norepinephrine, and serotonin levels—hormones that play a part in your ability to focus and feel mentally sharp. Exercise also stimulates the growth of new brain cells and helps prevent age-related decline.

In addition, exercise promotes the expression of brain-derived neurotrophic factor (BDNF), a protein that helps make new brain cells. As we age, our brain health declines. In fact, once you are in your twenties, your brain starts losing 10,000 brain cells a day! So we need all the help we can get. Physical activity is a natural way to increase BDNF, which protects the brain from deterioration, improves cognition, and can help ward off depression and anxiety.[6] BDNF also strengthens the connection between neurons, which boosts learning and memory.

Additionally, exercise helps with neurogenesis (i.e., creating new neurons) in the hippocampus, which is responsible for storing memory and learning.[7] Generating new neurons is one more cognitive benefit of exercise: when you work out your body, you also make your brain healthier!

8. Boost Your Mood

When you exercise, your body produces endorphins, like epinephrine and norepinephrine, which are natural mood lifters. Additionally, your body releases serotonin when you work out, which helps your brain regulate mood, sleep, and appetite. Movement also decreases overall stress and reduces immune system chemicals that can make mood disorders worse.

Many people find that exercise is a distraction from negative thoughts and emotions. It can help you feel a sense of accomplishment and confidence. For some, exercise is also an opportunity to connect with others—neighbors can walk together or friends can meet up at the gym. And because exercise helps you sleep better, it helps you wake up on the right side of the bed!

9. Enhance the Health of Your Skin

Many people use creams or formulas that promise to brighten their skin or increase their glow. An inexpensive way to achieve a similar effect is to do a good workout! When you exercise, blood flow increases throughout your body. Your blood then carries more oxygen and nutrients to all of the working cells throughout your body, including your skin. And it also carries waste products (like free radicals) *away* from your cells—decreasing toxins that cause damage to your skin and create an aging effect. So, not only does exercise increase blood flow to your skin, but it also helps protect your skin cells by increasing the production of natural antioxidants,[8] making your skin look fabulous without breaking the bank.

10. Live Longer

Studies show that exercise is a way to combat aging at a *cellular level*.[9] Our tightly packed DNA strands appear to shorten as we age. With each cell division, the protective end caps called *telomeres* (which normally protect the chromosome from damage) become shorter. Eventually, they become so short, the cell can no longer divide. This means our cells can't effectively do their job because they don't have as much DNA material to work with, which ultimately causes our cells to age. These same studies also determine that individuals who are more physically active have longer telomere lengths than sedentary participants. We don't know exactly why, but experts believe it's connected to decreased inflammation and oxidative stress. What we do know: longer telomeres help us age better.

What's the bottom line? Physical activity helps you live longer and healthier. Regular movement reduces many major mortality risk factors, such as diabetes, heart disease, stroke, and cancer. In fact, all-cause mortality is decreased by about 30–35 percent in physically active subjects compared to inactive subjects.[10] So if you like the idea of doing an around-the-world cruise in your retirement, or seeing your grandchildren graduate high-school, let this be a selling point for getting some exercise!

But just what type of movement qualifies as exercise? Should you simply try to get your heart rate up? Should you mainly focus on building muscle? First, let's discuss the specific kinds of movement your body needs to experience all the benefits listed here.

ELEMENTS OF A COMPLETE EXERCISE PROGRAM

One of my patients, Ben, is all about going to the gym and lifting weights. He always has been. He wants to look good, and building muscle has been his main focus of activity for many years. Unfortunately, lately, he's been feeling stiff and inflexible and has even put so much strain on his body that he needs shoulder surgery for a torn tendon.

Strength training certainly isn't bad; it's a key component of a balanced fitness program. However, as Ben experienced, it can imbalance the body when it's the *only* exercise modality you engage in.

Ben's story is not unique. Many people like him tend to focus on strength training to build muscle; others concentrate mainly on cardiovascular exercise because they want to lose weight. However, for an exercise program to be balanced and complete, we must include different types of movement. In this chapter, we'll put movement into the following categories:

♦ Aerobic

♦ Strength training

♦ Flexibility

♦ Core and balance

Let's consider why each type of movement is important for your cellular health.

Aerobic

Aerobic means "with oxygen," and aerobic activity conditions your heart. Therefore, your heart and lungs work together to bring oxygen to your muscles to help them burn fuel and move. You'll experience the greatest benefit to your body if you do your aerobic exercise throughout the week rather than being a weekend warrior. If you spread out your exercise, you'll experience the benefits of an increased metabolic rate throughout the week, whereas if you only work out on Saturday, you get that benefit through Sunday—but not necessarily beyond. Spreading out your exercise can also help prevent injury.

> **#CellCare:** The US Department of Health and Human Services recommends at least 150 minutes of moderate activity or 75 minutes of vigorous activity each week—that's only *21 minutes of moderate activity a day!*

Moderate aerobic activities include brisk walking, recreational swimming, doubles tennis, vinyasa yoga, water aerobics, and bicycling. Even yard work, house cleaning, and home repairs count!

Vigorous activities include running, swimming laps, jumping rope, HIIT workouts, and singles tennis. Depending on the type, dancing can be moderate or vigorous, and cycling can also fall under both categories.

The goal of aerobic training is to condition the heart to work better. Still, we also want to increase our ability to do more physical activity, whether it's an increase in duration, intensity, or both. Thus, aerobic training helps us both strengthen the heart and build endurance.

> **#CellCare:** Aerobic exercise will give you a burst of energy because it raises your heart rate and releases endorphins. For that reason, it is ideal to complete aerobic exercises at least three hours before bedtime so your body can rest; otherwise, it can disrupt your sleep.

Strength Training

Strength training, also known as resistance training, improves the strength of your major muscle groups. For example, while aerobic training strengthens the heart muscle, strength training reinforces your peripheral muscles, like your arms and legs, increasing your ability to perform certain activities. It can be done using weights or your body weight.

Strength training is recommended at least two days per week. The purpose is to make your muscles work harder than they usually do. So, if your muscles feel tired and are mildly sore after your workout, you're doing it right! The aim is to use as many major muscle groups as possible, training each group at least two times a week. This is why you hear people say, "I'm doing my upper back and chest today," or, "It's leg day." They're splitting up their workouts to focus on different major muscle groups.

> **#CellCare:** Strength training is recommended at least two days per week for each major muscle group.

When you are strength training, you want to do at least a single set of each exercise for about twelve to fifteen reps. The weight also has to be heavy enough to tire and damage your muscles so they can undergo repair. When I say "damage" in this context, I'm talking about a good type of trauma. The trauma that muscles experience in strength training is necessary to enter the repair phase to get stronger. Over time, you may want to increase the weights or reps to continue building strength.

Granted, you can over-traumatize your muscles if you don't include time for recovery. Ben, for example, was doing strength training every day. Even though he was alternating muscle groups to allow rest and repair between them, he was simply not providing enough recovery time for his body. Recovery time gives your muscles a chance to build themselves back up after the "trauma" of a good workout, and if you deny your muscles this time, they could get seriously injured.[11] A balanced exercise program will always include post-exercise recovery time. Whatever your level of physical activity, strength training can make you stronger and improve your mood, thanks to those mood-boosting endorphins.[12]

Flexibility

Flexibility exercises, or stretching, increase our range of motion, improve our posture, and increase blood flow to the muscles. This is an essential form of movement to incorporate alongside aerobic and strength training. If Ben had been interspersing stretching into his strength training routine regularly, the tightness and strain in his tendons may not have been as damaging.

The American Heart Association and other organizations don't have specific recommendations for stretching. As an integrative physician, I recommend stretching for thirty minutes, two times per week at a minimum. Stretching for five to ten minutes daily is even better. You can easily incorporate a shorter duration of stretching into your day by including it in your morning routine. For example, if you wake up stiff, this is a great way to loosen up your body. Alternatively, you can also stretch before bed—this is particularly helpful after a long day of sitting at a desk, which can aggravate muscles. Even when you don't feel motivated to do aerobic or strength exercises, you can still benefit from a good stretch.

#CellCare: Consider a five-minute stretch before you hop into the shower. You can do another five minutes before bed.

Maintaining your flexibility is an important means of keeping your youth. When older adults show signs of stiffness or decreased mobility, it's usually because they've lost flexibility; stretching can help you stay limber for longer. However, there's another key reason that stretching keeps you young: it fuels your fascia.

FLEXIBILITY FOR THE FASCIA

What is *fascia*? The easiest way to explain it is to think about Spider-Man. Spider-Man has a costume that wraps tightly around his entire frame, and it looks as though it's made out of many tightly woven webs. Essentially, that's what our fascia is like. It's an organ that forms a thin layer of tissue directly beneath our epidermis and encases our entire body. The fascia serves an important role in your body by acting as an information highway—it sends and receives messages between connective tissue and the rest of the body. It's made of cells, fibers, and ground substance.

♦ There are a handful of different **cells** in the fascia. *Fibroblasts* produce the collagen matrix for the body and respond to mechanical stimulation like compression and weight-bearing. The *adipocytes* provide padding and endocrine function. And the *macrophages* and *mast cells* help with inflammation and immune function.

♦ The **fibers** create the framework. *Collagen* provides the structure for the fascia, and everything else hangs on to it. *Elastin* makes the tissue flexible, and *reticulin* is the meshwork that supports organs.

♦ **Ground substance** is the fluid between the cells and fiber, composed of water (60–70 percent), protein, and glycosaminoglycans (GAGS). We often see the word hyaluronic acid (HA) in beauty products, and that happens to be one of our GAGs produced by fibroblasts. HA is like a sponge, soaking up water and supplying moisture to our body. You might have seen Eva Longoria on TV in a Loreal ad, touching her face and talking about how HA helps "plump skin and reduce wrinkles." Eva Longoria is onto something— but HA doesn't just impact the skin on your face; it affects your entire fascia.

We have fewer fibroblasts, less HA, and more fibers as we age. This results in a stiffer fascia, which causes toxin accumulation and decreased hydration. Some research also suggests that fibroblasts lose their functional identity in the sense that they stop producing collagen or HA the way they're supposed to and instead start behaving more like fat cells (a.k.a. adipocytes).[13] This is what causes your arms to "jiggle" or your facial skin to sag—our fibroblasts are having an identity crisis and our cells are not healing properly. But it also happens internally, in the walls of our blood vessels and organs. No thanks!

You can keep your fascia healthy by making good lifestyle choices. These include a plant-predominant diet that contains lots of antioxidants, good hydration, an active lifestyle, quality sleep, good posture, and reduced stress.

Why does fascia matter in terms of flexibility training? As we age, our fibroblasts decrease, and our bodies become stiffer and less elastic. We naturally lose hyaluronic acid, but we can lose even more if we don't move our tissues. Not moving your body clearly results in the "if you don't use it, you'll lose it" effect when it comes to the fascia. Not moving your body can cause the structures that hold your body together to weaken—everything gets saggy and loose.

Essentially, the firmness of your skin is determined by the quality of your fascia. Our skin doesn't look older as we age because we have *less* fascia; it's because the fascia has decreased in quality. The fascia becomes dehydrated, and the number of collagen-producing fibroblasts decreases. Some of these effects of aging are inevitable, but we can help our fascia maintain its optimal state by stretching and hydrating well. For example, stretching for ten minutes a day can ensure we keep our fibroblasts as peppy as possible, allowing us to stay relatively flexible. A "peppy" fibroblast can produce HA (attention, Eva Longoria) and collagen for the entire body. Hydration is also key: water makes up about 60–70 percent of your ground substance. Hydration and stretching also work together: stretching the body helps to hydrate your fascia, because it increases your circulation.

Core and Balance Exercises

Core exercises improve the muscles of your pelvis, lower back, hips, and abdomen—your body's core. It's important to strengthen these muscles because they provide stability and balance for the body during our daily activities.

Consider the movements your body undergoes as you pick up a small child: it requires bending down, lateral spine movement, pulling the child back up, and then holding that child mainly on one side of your body. All of this requires tremendous action in your core. Or imagine bending down to empty the trunk of your car, lifting heavy suitcases or grocery bags out while your spine is still bent. Think of joining a game of pick-up basketball, soccer, or volleyball—those quick shifts of your body weight all use your core. We use and rely on our core muscles all of the time.

Without a strong core, your back and hips can begin to feel strained when you do these everyday movements. However, a strong core will help you move efficiently, maintain good posture, sustain balance and stability, and prevent injury.

Balance training should also be incorporated into your day, especially as you get older; it's effective in preventing falls and other injuries and will also help improve your mobility.

Core and balance training is often an afterthought in our exercise routines, despite its importance. I recommend incorporating core and balance with your other exercises for five to ten minutes daily. With our busy schedules, doing a few minutes every day is more manageable than finding time for an entire core workout, especially if you're already doing aerobics and strength training during the week. For example, holding a plank for sixty seconds every day will build your core better than cramming in a hundred sit-ups over the weekend.

#CellCare: The best way to build a strong core is with daily exercise—even just a few minutes per day. Consider doing a plank every time the opening credits appear during your favorite show.

Your body needs all of these types of movement to maintain balance and homeostasis. But, like Ben, you can sustain injury if your routine is imbalanced.

Here's a great synopsis of all the amazing benefits that come from regularly moving your body, courtesy of the American College of Sports Medicine:[14]

- Significantly improve overall health

- Decrease depression as effectively as medications or therapy

- Reduce risk of heart disease by 40 percent

- Reduce incidence of high blood pressure and diabetes by almost 50 percent

- Reduce risk of colon cancer by over 60 percent

- Reduce mortality and risk of recurrent breast cancer by almost 50 percent

- Reduce risk of developing Alzheimer's by one-third

Basically, exercise makes you smarter, stronger, and healthier for life. But before we end the discussion on exercise, there's one more key aspect of your body's movement to discuss: your breath.

That's right—you need to learn how to breathe efficiently.

Breath is one other aspect of movement that might seem insignificant, but this couldn't be further from the truth. Given that all of your muscles require oxygen to function optimally, your body needs plenty of it to fully thrive. That means all of us can benefit from learning a few pointers on improving our breathing.

THE SCIENCE OF BREATH

The majority of us inhale and exhale shallowly, breathing only into the upper part of our lungs. When you breathe, if you only feel your chest rises and fall, you're not breathing deeply. Shallow (or thoracic) breathing is not the most optimal way to breathe because less air intake puts more stress on the body. Shallow breathing causes stress and stress causes shallow breathing—a cycle that can trigger health issues and compromise our immune system. In addition, when you breathe improperly, you aren't getting adequate oxygen and nutrients to your body. As a result, you aren't effectively exhaling carbon dioxide (CO_2) out of your body, which means more toxic CO_2 remains, causing cellular damage.

Ideally, when you breathe, you should use your diaphragm to bring oxygen down into the deeper part of your lungs. You'll know you are using your diaphragm if you feel your stomach expand and contract when breathing: that's a sign you're breathing deeply into your belly. The *diaphragm* is a parachute-shaped skeletal muscle that sits between the thoracic and abdominal cavities. It contracts and flattens when we inhale, and as we exhale, it relaxes, pushing air out of the lungs. Proper breathing requires using the diaphragm because it facilitates the full inflation of the lungs and helps expel carbon dioxide on the exhale. Most singers, actors, musicians, and athletes have learned this trick so that they can optimize their vocal output and their body's endurance. Proper breathing also means breathing in through your nose, which acts as a filter and humidifier. The latest research has also demonstrated that there is a direct link between nasal breathing and cognitive function.[15]

When you learn to breathe properly, your movements take less effort and energy because you're effectively meeting your body's demand for oxygen. The decrease in the effort also helps to slow your breathing rate, which means your heart doesn't have to work as hard.

RITUALS FOR MOVEMENT

By now, you probably see the incredible benefits of movement, so creating a ritual around activity that is sustainable for your lifestyle should be a priority. If you're just beginning, start with the most fun activity for you. If you are advanced, consider techniques to create a balanced routine. Let's start with optimizing our breath in order to reap the benefits of any movement ritual we choose.

4-7-8 Breath

One of my mentors, Dr. Andrew Weil, introduced me to this breathing technique. I remember sitting in the classroom, watching him take an inhale and exhale with a swoosh sound. He described it as a "natural tranquilizer for the nervous system." Here's how to practice this technique:

◆ For a count of four, inhale through your nose with your lips closed.

◆ For a count of seven, hold your breath.

◆ For a count of eight, exhale completely through your mouth, making a whoosh sound.

◆ This makes one cycle. Repeat for a total of four cycles.

By exhaling longer than you inhale, you activate the vagus nerve. Remember, as discussed in Chapter Four, the vagus nerve is a two-way communication between your gut and your brain, and also happens to be the longest nerve in the body. Deep breathing triggers the vagus nerve to send the message to your brain that it's time to shift into a relaxed, parasympathetic state. By focusing on your breath for those specific counts, you can remind yourself to breathe deeply and use your diaphragm. This not only helps you oxygenate adequately but can also help you calm heightened emotions and decrease your level of stress.

Diaphragmatic Breathing

We've already discussed the importance of efficient breathing and using the diaphragm. To see if you're breathing correctly, place one hand on your chest and one on your belly, then breathe in through your nose and out of your mouth. If the hand on your chest rises, you are doing shallow breathing. If the hand on your belly rises, you are doing belly breathing (which we want). Diaphragmatic breathing can strengthen your core muscles and lower your blood pressure. Here's how to practice this technique:

- Lay down on your back in a comfortable position.

- Place one hand in the middle of your chest and place your other hand on your abdomen, just below the rib cage.

- Inhale through the nose slowly, drawing the breath to the stomach (this is where the stomach should push upward against the hand while your chest remains still).

- Exhale through pursed lips as the stomach falls downward.

- Repeat three to four times a day for five minutes.

With practice, diaphragmatic breathing will become your natural way of breathing and you will no longer need to lie down to do it. Studies have found that this type of breathing can lower cortisol levels, thereby alleviating stress and helping your respiratory cells function optimally.[16]

Straw Breathing (Pursed Lip Breathing)

In five minutes, you can quickly increase feelings of calm and relaxation with this technique, which can be done with or without a straw. Ultimately, it leads to more air getting into the lungs, the lungs working more efficiently, and the airways being open longer. Here's how to practice this technique:

♦ Inhale through your nose for two seconds.

♦ Next, purse the lips and exhale, pushing the air out through a drinking straw (or, if you do not have a straw, imagine that you're blowing out candles on a cake).

♦ Finally, exhale slowly through the pursed lips for four to six seconds.

I recommend you do this exercise for five minutes, twice a day. You can keep a straw in your bag and do this exercise whenever you're feeling anxious.

#**CellCare:** Once you've mastered some of these breathing techniques, you may want to explore these more advanced practices: alternate nostril breathing (*nadi shodhana*), box breathing, Lion's breath (*simhasana*), or the more advanced *kapalabhati* breath.

Let's now turn to the rest of your body. I will leave you to choose your favorite conventional aerobic and resistance exercises, while I introduce you to some forms of movements you may not have considered. These are some of my favorites.

YOUR BODY IS MEANT TO MOVE

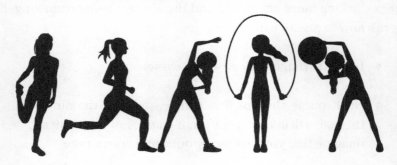

Yoga as Medicine

Vinyasa yoga is the best example of aerobic, strength, flexibility, and core training, all rolled into one activity. We live in a demanding, stressful world, and this practice will benefit anyone and everyone because of the comprehensive ways it helps the mind and body. Yoga can be a combination of asana (postures), pranayama (breathing), and meditation. It helps train you in proper breathing and balances your nervous system. One researcher writes, "We underestimate the power of aligning our breath with movement, but the effects can be transformative. Studies show that yogic practices enhance muscular strength and body flexibility, promote and improve respiratory and cardiovascular function, promote recovery from and treatment of addiction, reduce stress, anxiety, depression, and chronic pain, improve sleep patterns, and enhance overall wellbeing and quality of life."[17]

In fact, because of the tremendous impact I see yoga making in my patients' lives (and my own!) I consider it to be a form of medicine. Even better, research informs us that yoga may be superior to other forms of exercise in its positive effect on mood and anxiety.[18] And, considering that yoga postures increase GABA levels (the neurotransmitter that increases relaxation and alleviates pain), there's no reason not to roll out the yoga mat!

My favorite yoga ritual is **Sun Salutations**. This sequence of yoga poses aligns your breath with your movement. You can find video tutorials on how to do Sun Salutations at yogamedicine.com. Consider this a private date with yourself in which you go through a series of yoga postures to welcome the day, stretch your body, focus your mind, and strengthen your muscles.

INHALE, EXHALE, REPEAT

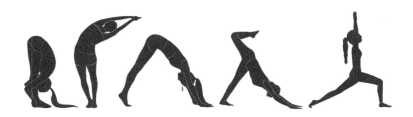

Five Tibetans Practice

The Five Tibetans Practice is a rejuvenation practice that's 2,500 years old. It's as if you're floating through a meditative dance, repeating a brief pattern twenty-one times. There are five movements in the sequence: twirling, leg raises, dynamic camel, moving tabletop, and downward dog to upward dog.[19] A quick YouTube tutorial will help you get started and provide guidance.

The Tibetans consider this practice the "fountain of youth" of exercises, helping people turn back the clock on aging. This practice is based on the body's energy and can improve your balance. Consider incorporating this as part of your flexibility ritual.

Abdominal Activation

A 2020 study from the *International Journal of Environmental Research and Public Health* found that when the *abdominal hollowing method* (AHM; the activation and pulling in of the navel) was employed in a traditional plank position, it proved to be an effective strategy for increasing overall abdominal activity, particularly in your internal and external obliques (i.e., the "six pack" muscles).[20] Small form adjustments, like the AHM technique, can have major body benefits. When performing a plank, activate your deep abdominal muscles by pulling in your navel. If you've been struggling to strengthen your core or get a more toned physique, this would be a great ritual to try.

Myofascial Release

Earlier in this chapter, we talked about the fascia; *myofascial* specifically relates to the muscle and fascia connection—which is often an area where we carry knots and trigger-point pain. Myofascial release is a relatively simple practice that can help increase your flexibility and alleviate pain; it's used in massage therapy, but you can also do it on your own. Myofascial release involves using a tool with a round surface—like a ball or a foam roller—to put pressure between the muscle and the fascia. This pressure provides hydration and nutrients to areas of tension. When areas of the body get tight, use myofascial release to apply pressure to those areas to ease pain and restore normal blood flow and function.

Myofascial release can be a welcome addition to your nighttime ritual. For example, while watching TV, use a foam roller or myofascial release balls to release tension in your legs, back, neck, and arms. Myofascial release can be done on literally any part of the body—wherever you feel tension. The technique can include compression, rolling, rocking, and lengthening to apply hydration to the tissues. Rather than going to bed with pain or tension, myofascial release will help your body repair the strain you might experience in daily life.

Gratitude Walk

Take a ten-minute "thank you" walk. Consider all the things around you that you can give thanks for—the beauty that you see, the slant of the sunlight, the wind through the trees. Slowing down allows you the chance to breathe deeper and take in your surroundings. Call to mind the people you love and the tasks that you were able to accomplish that day. Even the fact that you're capable of walking is a reason to give thanks. Entering into this grateful frame of mind will help put you in a relaxed, parasympathetic state, as the movement helps your circulation and produces endorphins. The result will be a potent mood lift, a boost to your immune system, and better circadian rhythm to sleep soundly.

Rhythms of Nature

Shirin-Yoku translates to "forest bathing." The practice doesn't mean skinny dipping in a forest stream, but rather "bathing yourself" in the sensory sensations of the forest. It was developed in Japan in the '80s and has become a part of healing in Japanese medicine. You can even consider it a cross between fitness and mindfulness. Researchers found that spending time amongst the trees creates neuropsychological effects that can boost the immune system and reduce the stress hormone cortisol.[21] This type of nature therapy can be applied to address modern-day stress, including "technostress," the stress of always being connected via your phone, email, and social media accounts.[22] You don't need a forest to try this activity; you can simply take a leisurely walk on a local trail. Here's how to practice this technique:

♦ To begin, leave your phone behind (or at least turn off your device), so you can be present in the experience.

♦ Next, leave your expectations behind and allow your body to wander wherever it wants.

♦ Take time to pause and notice your surroundings— the leaves, the smells, the sensations beneath your feet.

♦ Find a spot to sit and take in your surroundings— the sounds of the air, the birds chirping, the colors, nature all around you. Try to avoid thinking about your to-do lists.

♦ Lastly, if you do this activity with others, opt not to talk until the end of the walk, where you can then discuss your experience.

♦ Stay as long as you can and gradually build-up to the recommended two hours.

Motivational Music

Have you ever heard a song that made you want to move your body? Some of the most successful athletes have a "get pumped" playlist, like Serena Williams and Roger Federer. Creating a playlist can be one of the best things for your workout routine to enhance physical performance.[23] You may even create three playlists:

♦ A pre-workout playlist to get you pumped on your drive to the gym.

♦ A workout playlist to keep you motivated.

♦ A post-workout playlist to help you relax after completing your activity.

There is more than hype to a playlist—it can activate certain parts of your brain that create beneficial effects. For example, listening to music can enhance the frontal lobe, which is responsible for thinking and decision-making. In addition, music may increase new brain cells in the hippocampus, creating new neurons for improving memory. That's why playlists can stir up memories of certain seasons in your life. Music can also increase the body's production of antibodies and decrease cortisol production, enhancing your immune system.[24] In short, music can make you stronger, smarter, boost your immune system, and enhance your overall wellbeing.[25] Think of music as an invitation to move your body and promote cellular longevity.

Clothes, Shoes, Bag, Go

It's easy for us to find reasons not to go to the gym or do a workout. That's because without planning, it probably won't happen. Maybe that's where you are right now: struggling to find the motivation to even plan a workout. If that's you, that's okay. At the top of your list, the ritual may simply be to gather the gear you need to get to that next step. That might look like indulging in a new workout outfit to help you get motivated. Or organizing your workout clothes like you do your work outfits. Lay everything out where you'll see it first thing in the morning, and have it ready to go. Then, when you see that outfit, you may feel inspired to put it on and move your body just a little.

If you eliminate unnecessary decisions around your workout routine, such as what you're going to wear or what sort of exercise you're going to do, then you leave yourself only one decision to make: "What physical activity does my body need today?" When all the other decisions are already in place, you're more likely to use that momentum to get the workout your body needs most.

Activity with Intention

Having purposeful physical activity is important, but there are also ways you can incorporate regular movement into your day without feeling overwhelmed by the prospect of going to the gym.

◆ Do squats while waiting for the coffee to brew.

◆ Try balancing on one foot while brushing your teeth.

- ◆ If there are stairs, use them instead of the elevator.

- ◆ Park farther away and walk more.

- ◆ Gather with friends for a hike (rather than around a meal).

- ◆ Use resistance bands during commercial breaks, rather than fast forwarding on your DVR.

By incorporating just one or two of these rituals, you can help your body become stronger, energized, and more flexible. All of these practices will also provide you with a noticeable mood lift and decrease your stress.

Moving your body doesn't need to require an expensive membership—all you need is a plan, an intention, and about ten minutes to start!

Reflect on Your #CellCare

Using these guiding questions, take a moment to build self-awareness and reflect on movement in your life:

♦ What are your motivators for exercise? What inspires you to be active? How does movement make you feel?

♦ What are you doing regularly that gets you moving? Do you incorporate cardio, strength, flexibility, balance, and core training in your week?

♦ Do you prefer to exercise in groups or alone? Do you prefer for your mind to be engaged while exercising (i.e., music, audiobooks, podcasts)?

♦ Do you have an intentional breathing practice?

♦ Do you have any obstacles to engaging in movement and physical activity? What are possible solutions to your obstacles, and how can you overcome them?

DESIGN YOUR WELLBEING

In the space below, note your thoughts about the art of movement. First, note what movement you are doing now and what you want to incorporate in the future. Next, write down why you want to do that activity. Then, name a ritual you may want to incorporate into your life and how often you would like to do it.

6

RESTORATIVE RECOVERY

"Tired minds don't plan well. Sleep first, plan later."

~ WALTER REISCH, AUSTRIAN SCREENWRITER

KYLE, A POPULAR EIGHTEEN-YEAR-OLD BOY, BECAME MY patient during his first year of college. He was having trouble keeping up with his classes. He felt tired in the morning and rundown through the afternoon. He drank coffee and Red Bull multiple times a day, stayed up late to study, and often had pizzas delivered to his dorm room at 2:00 a.m.

Kyle was a pre-med student, so there was tremendous pressure to keep his GPA at a certain level. However, when he got his grades for the last semester, they were mediocre at best. At that moment, he panicked. Kyle felt like he studied all the time, so he couldn't understand his poor academic performance.

Even though Kyle was logging many hours in the library, he wasn't absorbing much of the information due to his lack of sleep. Sleep is necessary for the brain to process and store information (more on that soon). So he was stuck in a vicious cycle: he felt exhausted from not sleeping, tried to compensate for the lack of sleep with caffeine, and then—when he did sleep—he did so restlessly because the caffeine had him wired.

Kyle was also trying to put on weight and build muscle, but he was not seeing his desired results. Once again, the issue was Kyle's lack of *quality* sleep. He worked out often, but the lack of sleep didn't allow his growth hormone to kick in. His poor sleep wasn't just affecting his energy and academic performance; it also affected his athletic performance.

Kyle's studying wasn't the only reason he stayed awake late. He also texted his friends, played games on his computer, and took advantage of the freshman life. I asked if his friends were sending important messages in the middle of the night. He grinned sheepishly and told me *no*—usually, their conversations could wait until the next day.

When I explained to Kyle all the ways that his lack of sleep was negatively affecting both his short- and long-term goals, he was shocked. He had no idea that sleep quality played a significant role in his success as a student and athlete. Especially since he was living in the company of other college students, Kyle assumed it was normal to pull all-nighters, stay up late partying, and survive on caffeine. However, when he began to understand how much more successful he might be with a few extra hours of shut-eye, he was ready to make changes.

After our conversations, Kyle started to make small changes that felt sustainable for a college freshman, starting with an earlier bedtime. He also changed some of his sleep hygiene: no caffeine after 4:00 p.m., no screen time within a half-hour of when he planned to sleep, and he laid off the partying, except on weekends. I was not surprised when Kyle gleefully told me that his grades started improving, even though he hadn't changed his studying efforts. Over a number of consultations, Kyle's small, incremental changes and intentional rituals made a big impact on his academic performance and overall health.

We often treat sleep like a routine. We work or play until we can't anymore, and then we grudgingly sleep so we can go on to continue the business of living. But sleep isn't just a routine—it's a dynamic process that plays a vital role in our wellbeing.

THE GIFT OF SLEEP

Sleep is one of the most important gifts we can give to our bodies, but we often undermine the quality of our sleep with poor lifestyle habits. That's a big deal: all sleep is not created equal, and the main benefits of sleep occur in deep sleep. We spend one-third of our lifetime sleeping, so by increasing the quality of our rest, we can ensure we're getting the most out of the two-thirds of the day we are awake.

A lack of quality sleep can have many consequences for your brain, body, and wellbeing. Insufficient sleep means your brain can't optimally function because neurotransmitters and neurons cannot rest or regenerate.[1] If your brain cells can't rest, your "happy hormones" are affected—that's why sleep deprivation makes you cranky!

Numerous studies have shown a lack of sleep can affect memory recall and decrease your cognitive performance—just think of Kyle's struggles. Certain stages of sleep are needed to regenerate neurons within the cerebral cortex. Other stages of sleep appear to be used to form new memories and generate new synaptic connections.[2] Those are the connections between your brain cells, and they are what enable you to process emotions, build memories, and repair tissue. Basically, the synaptic connections are what makes your brain work! And sleep is integral for all of it.

Poor-quality sleep can even cause some neurons in the brain to malfunction. If your neurons aren't functioning correctly, it affects behavior and can hurt your academic or professional performance. What's the ultimate effect of our compromised cognitive performance? Studies have proven that lack of sleep harms long-term and working memory, attention, high-order executive function, and various decision-making processes.[3] In other words, when you don't sleep well, you're not thinking clearly.

And what about the effects on your body? Restful sleep leads to the production of your growth hormones, body tissue repair, and improved immune function. That means when you *don't* sleep well, your muscles can't build, your body struggles more to heal itself, and you struggle to fend off disease. Over time, these adverse effects can lead to chronic health issues.

There are also psychological impacts as well. Insufficient sleep leads to elevated stress levels. You've probably experienced that high stress firsthand if you've ever been irritable or weepy when tired. Sleep is necessary to regenerate the brain so it continues to function normally.[4] Research also shows that sleep loss makes it difficult to "look on the bright side." When we're functioning from a place of fatigue, we have stronger reactions to stressful situations, whereas ample sleep helps us respond better to positive and negative situations.[5] If you often find yourself feeling overwhelmed, focusing on your sleep ritual might make a big difference in your wellbeing.

Those are some of the negative impacts of not getting enough sleep, but I find it even more compelling to look at the *benefits* we experience *from* sleep. Let's look at a comprehensive list of all the gifts we experience when we allow our bodies to deeply rest:

♦ **Bigger muscles:** During deep sleep, your body releases growth hormones. The more your body wants to grow, the more sleep you're going to need. For instance, babies sleep for sixteen to eighteen hours a day because they're in a major growth phase. As adults, the growth hormone no longer spurs on height, but it does play a role in keeping your muscles healthy, improving your bone density, and reducing your body fat.

♦ **Smarter brain:** Information is consolidated in the brain, which means everything you're trying to learn during the day has a chance to stick after a good night's sleep. A recent study published in the journal *Sleep* showed that ample sleep restores clarity and performance by actively refining cortical plasticity.[6]

♦ **Cleaner system:** During sleep, toxins are removed from the *glymphatic* system, which you can think of as your brain's custodial staff. The glymphatic system uses a network of small blood vessels formed by *astroglial* cells to flush out cellular trash in the brain, much like a plumbing system. Importantly, researchers have found "the glymphatic system functions mainly during sleep and is largely disengaged during wakefulness."[7] In other words, when you don't sleep as well, your brain custodians aren't effectively eliminating the cellular trash from your brain. The effects become apparent in diminished cognitive abilities, behavior, and judgment.[8]

♦ **A tidied mind:** The glymphatic system not only clears toxins *out* of your brain, it also tidies up, helping to distribute important compounds that help your cognition, such as amino acids, glucose, lipids, and neurotransmitters. The combination of clearing *out* the toxic waste and distributing these helpful compounds enables your brain to maintain optimal function.

♦ **Better memory:** During sleep, the brain continues to function; it's not turned off. The rest of the body slows down and rests, but the brain is still active as it essentially recharges itself and consolidates the important information from the day. This is why sleep is so important for your memory.

♦ **Greater wellbeing:** Sleep regulates your metabolism and reduces mental fatigue, meaning when you wake up, you feel rested and refreshed. On the other hand, chronic sleep deprivation is associated with serious emotional challenges.

♦ **Improved health:** Sleep also affects your immune

system and mental health. People who sleep well have an easier time fighting off viruses, like the common cold. They also tend to experience greater psychological wellbeing. When you're tired, you generally have less energy, are more irritable, and are less focused.

#CellCare: How much sleep does your body need, and does that change as you age? Here are some specific numbers provided by the American Academy of Sleep Medicine:

- Infants: 12–16 hours[9]

- Toddlers: 11–14 hours

- Preschool age: 10–13 hours

- School age: 9–12 hours

- Teenagers: 8–10 hours[10]

- Adults: 7 or more hours[11]

At the end of this chapter, I will provide strategies to help optimize your sleeping hours. But before we go there, let's learn how sleep works.

THE SCIENCE OF SLEEP

There are two internal biological mechanisms that work together to usher in and regulate your sleep: your circadian rhythm and your sleep–wake homeostasis. Additionally, by learning about your brain waves and heart rate variability, you can better understand how to optimize your sleep.

Circadian Rhythm

Your *circadian rhythm* is your body's internal clock, based on a twenty-four-hour cycle. Relying on light changes in our environment, it can regulate alertness and sleepiness. Although we associate it most with our sleep–wake cycle, your circadian rhythm impacts much more than that. It regulates several physiologic responses in your body, such as your body temperature, blood pressure, when to release certain hormones, when to metabolize your food, and so on, in addition to your sleep and wakefulness. Your circadian rhythm is affected by your daily patterns of sleep, along with other elements of your lifestyle such as the timing of your meals, your technology habits, and your exercise routine.

How does this work? There's an area of the brain with thousands of cells that all receive information related to your circadian rhythm when exposed to light. Those thousands of cells live in an area called the *suprachiasmatic nucleus (SCN)* of the hypothalamus, and this part of the brain is essentially the circadian "pacemaker." Using the information they're getting about light, these cells collectively inform the rest of your body when it's time to be awake and when it's time to sleep. When your body is exposed to daylight, physiologic changes occur that signal it's time to be awake; specifically, your body starts producing cortisol, which makes you feel alert and awake, with levels high in the morning. When it's dark, on the other hand, your body recognizes that it's time for sleep. The hypothalamus signals to the pineal gland to produce melatonin, your sleepy hormone. It also makes the chemical GABA (gamma-aminobutyric acid), an amino acid that works as a neurotransmitter to your brain, associated with sleep, muscle relaxation, and sedation. The result: your body starts making the transition to sleep.

> **#CellCare:** The health of your cells is connected to the health of your sleep. And—because your circadian rhythm (using molecular feedback loops) is affected by your environment—your environment ends up having a direct impact on your sleep and therefore your cellular health.
>
> What's the take away? Optimize your circadian rhythm, and you'll be optimizing your #CellCare.

Many of us create lots of confusion for our melatonin-inducing hypothalamus by manipulating our light exposure. For example, we might work in a dark office during the day and then expose ourselves to blue light at night via cell phones, TV screens, and other bright lights. Unfortunately, this circadian confusion can mean our bodies don't know to produce melatonin once we finally lay down to rest. This is hard on our bodies: we often get low-quality sleep, contributing to health issues.

As much as possible, use your body's sensitivity to light to train your circadian rhythm. Ideally, you should expose yourself to sunlight when you wake and sleep in a dark room. Medications, stress, alcohol, and inconsistent sleeping habits can negatively impact your circadian rhythms. Later in this chapter, we'll discuss how you can support your body's circadian rhythm through avoiding sleep sabotage and prioritizing sleep hygiene. When our rituals align with our natural circadian rhythms, our bodies generally function the way they should.

Sleep–Wake Homeostasis

The second internal biological mechanism that helps usher in sleep is your *sleep–wake homeostasis*. This process keeps track of how much sleep you need; it's the reason you might feel the need for a midday nap if you're not getting sufficient rest at night or the reason you yawn during dinner if you stayed up until 2:00 a.m. the night before. The homeostatic sleep drive works via the production of an inhibitory neurotransmitter called adenosine, which makes you sleepy. The longer you're awake, the more adenosine you have collected in your brain. In normal conditions, the build-up of adenosine signals the body to rest.

When you fight your body's inclination toward sleepiness, your sleep–wake cycle can get out of alignment. That can make it a bigger challenge to get quality sleep later on. Your body's natural awareness can be improved by practicing good sleep hygiene to ensure your body gets the sleep it needs.

#**CellCare:** Your afternoon caffeine intake blocks the action of adenosine in the brain, therefore increasing wakefulness. You might think this is helpful in the short term, but actually, this interferes with your natural sleep–wake cycle, which can end up hindering your restful sleep at night; you're better off taking a power nap.

Brain Waves

Brain waves describe electrochemical activity that happen in your neurons. You have five different kinds of brain waves, and two are key for sleep:

Your **gamma** brain waves occur at the highest frequency, during your brain's peak activity. This is when your brain is literally receiving electrical bursts of high-level information, such as when you're learning something new that you're incredibly interested in. It's a place of creativity and enhanced cognition. **Beta** waves are where most of us live: they occur during our normal waking state, when we're alert and doing our "daily hustle." Beta waves would occur for students learning in school, or professionals engaged in a meeting. It's our problem-solving state when we're engaged and attentive—however, keeping yourself in a beta stage of mind for too long can zap your energy and lead to burn out. **Alpha** waves occur when we're relaxed. Often, your eyes are closed, like in a state of meditation; you might be reading a book or doing a calming yoga class. Your stress is lower and you have the ability to focus and think clearly.

BRAIN WAVES

GAMMA

Insight, heightened perception, and peak focus

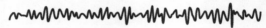

BETA

Engagement, alertness, and problem-solving

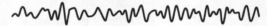

ALPHA

Reflection, relaxation, and visualization

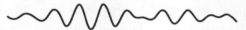

THETA

Flow state, dreaming, and meditation

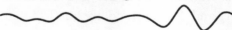

DELTA

Deep, restorative, preparative sleep

The final two brain waves are key for understanding how to get quality sleep. **Theta** waves describe your "autopilot" mode; think of how you operate while taking a shower or driving a familiar route. Theta waves are also present during deep meditation, day dreaming, light sleep, and REM sleep. In this state, our brains are able to rest, process emotions, and rejuvenate their creativity. Think of theta as your brain's "second gear."

First gear then, would be your **delta** waves, which occur at the lowest frequency. This is where your brain is at during *deep* sleep, and it's during this delta wave state that your body is reducing cortisol, rolling back the clock on your aging, and restoring and repairing your cells.

> **#CellCare:** You can manipulate your brain waves for better mental health with a regular meditation practice, which increases your relaxed brain alpha waves. The previously mentioned breathing practices in Chapter Five also boost alpha waves. Besides helping us feel relaxed, this boost of alpha waves can act as a natural antidepressant by promoting serotonin release.

Heart Rate Variability as an Indicator of Sleep Quality

One of the main indicators used to track the quality of your sleep via sleep trackers is your heart rate variability. Contrary to what many may think, the heart doesn't beat at a steady rate. It fluctuates from beat to beat. This is known as *heart rate variability* or HRV. Our HRV is controlled by the autonomic nervous system (i.e., your sympathetic and parasympathetic responses, discussed in Chapter Two), meaning it's involuntary. HRV is different than your heart rate. Whereas your heart rate measures the speed of your heart's beats, commonly known as your pulse, your HRV measures the variability *between* beats. This number indicates how quickly we recover and bounce back from stressful events: essentially, it's a symbol of our heart's resilience.

HRV is typically monitored during sleep, and the numbers can tell us something about our cardiac health. A *low* HRV would mean your heart rate struggles to respond quickly to external circumstances; a *higher* HRV would suggest your body has a strong ability to tolerate stressful events and recover from accumulated stress.

Interestingly enough, HRV also seems closely linked to the quality of sleep, although scientists are still learning why that might be. People who get low-quality sleep also usually have decreased HRV numbers, but a higher HRV number typically indicates better quality sleep.[12] Higher HRV can also be a sign of youthful physiology[13,] and less mental stress.[14] As we age, our average HRV numbers typically decrease.[15]

Since HRV is linked to the balance between your sympathetic (fight and flight) response and your parasympathetic (rest and digest) response, it can also be a good indicator of your overall wellbeing and used as a gauge to determine how healthy you are. For instance, if your average sleeping HRV is low for your age, that can be a sign of premature aging. In addition, many of the rituals we discuss in this book can help you increase your HRV.

#CellCare: Here are ways to help increase your HRV:

♦ **Stick to a consistent sleep schedule.** Go to bed at the same time daily and wake up at the same time daily.

♦ **Get natural light exposure.** Open the curtains, or better yet, get outside in the morning.

♦ **Exercise regularly.** This is going to be one of the best ways to improve your HRV.[16]

♦ **Do mind–body exercises.** Activities such as yoga or Tai Chi help balance the sympathetic and parasympathetic nervous system, therefore impacting HRV.[17]

♦ **Engage in effective breathing.** Remember the differential breathing rituals I mentioned previously—these controlled breathing techniques can positively impact your HRV.[18]

♦ **Develop regular eating patterns.** The time of your food intake can impact your HRV, so having regular eating patterns can help your circadian rhythm and ultimately your HRV.

♦ **Take cold showers.** This one may not be at the top of your list, but if you have already included everything else, this is yet another way to expose your body to cold thermogenesis to stimulate the vagus nerve, which in turn stimulates the parasympathetic system and your HRV.

SLEEP STAGES

While we sleep, our brain goes through several stages, during which key biological processes happen. To some degree, most people know that there's a difference between genuinely restorative sleep and poor-quality sleep. We say things like, "I slept so well last night," or "I was tossing and turning all night long." The difference is real: truly restorative sleep goes through five complete stages, whereas shallow sleep may skim the top and only go through two or three. Our bodies require deep sleep to experience the most therapeutic effects.

The two fundamental phases of sleep are non-rapid eye movement (NREM) and rapid eye movement (REM), during which specific brainwaves and neuronal activity occur. Within the NREM phase, there are additional stages that take us from shallow sleep into deep sleep. Our body cycles through these two phases four to five times each night, with each complete cycle lasting around 90 to 120 minutes.

THE STAGES OF SLEEP

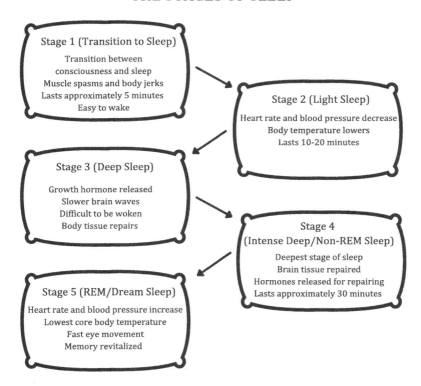

Stage 1 (Transition to Sleep)

Transition between
consciousness and sleep
Muscle spasms and body jerks
Lasts approximately 5 minutes
Easy to wake

Stage 2 (Light Sleep)

Heart rate and blood pressure decrease
Body temperature lowers
Lasts 10-20 minutes

Stage 3 (Deep Sleep)

Growth hormone released
Slower brain waves
Difficult to be woken
Body tissue repairs

Stage 4
(Intense Deep/Non-REM Sleep)

Deepest stage of sleep
Brain tissue repaired
Hormones released for repairing
Lasts approximately 30 minutes

Stage 5 (REM/Dream Sleep)

Heart rate and blood pressure increase
Lowest core body temperature
Fast eye movement
Memory revitalized

NREM: Stages 1 through 4

In **Stage 1**, we cross over from wakefulness to sleep. It's a short period, lasting only a few minutes. Sometimes, you might experience muscle spasms or jerks in this phase as your body begins to transition You can be easily woken from noise disturbances.

Stage 2 (light sleep) lasts between 10 and 20 minutes. In this stage, your breathing and heartbeat begin to slow down, your muscles relax further, and your body temperature lowers. Your brainwaves also start to slow from their wakeful daytime pattern, and your eye movements slow or stop. During this stage, your brain also experiences cognitive bursts of electrical activity, which improve your memory and learning abilities. These effects can help you feel refreshed and more alert after a short nap.

In **Stage 3 (deep sleep)** you transition even further into sleep, and it will be tough to wake you. This is when you start to see the significant benefits of sleep kick in as your pituitary gland releases growth hormone, the glymphatic system clears out toxins, and your memory and learning consolidate. Tissue growth and repair also takes place in this stage.

Insufficient time in Stage 3 means we don't experience the restorative benefits of deep sleep. In fact, my patient Kyle wasn't experiencing success with his late-night study sessions because he likely remained in a mostly shallow state of sleep, which meant his brain was not consolidating what he learned. His poor-quality sleep also meant he wasn't building new muscle mass, because his tissue wasn't getting much of a chance at repairing itself after his work outs.

Deep sleep is the "holy grail" we want to aim for when improving your sleep rituals since it's the stage that offers the most benefits for your body and mind.

In **Stage 4 (intense deep sleep)**, you experience your deepest sleep and the benefits that occur during Stage 3 continue. Whereas you started to experience body tissue repair in Stage 3, the repair goes even further in Stage 4, during which hormones are released to repair your brain tissue. In this stage of intense deep sleep, the brain will slow to its lowest levels. This is your "do not disturb" mode, where if you are woken, you will feel disoriented.

REM: Stage 5

REM (rapid eye movement) is **Stage 5** and occurs about 90 minutes after falling asleep, lasting for about 10 to 15 minutes. This is when you're most likely to dream. However, even though your mind is incredibly active during REM sleep, your body movements are temporarily paralyzed. Your arms and legs won't move, but your breathing, heart rate, and blood pressure rise. They function at the same rate as if you were awake, which is one reason why dreams can feel so real. You are in action within the dream, and your mind believes you are moving; in fact, that's likely why you experience the rapid eye movement that characterizes REM sleep. Luckily, even while the involuntary functions of the body increase, your voluntary actions won't; the temporary paralysis keeps you safe under your covers and prevents you from acting out your dream.

Significant emotional benefits come during REM sleep. The *dream rebound theory* suggests that dreams may help you process your emotions from the day or express emotions that are otherwise suppressed in your conscious state.[19] Emotions are linked to certain parts of the brain, including the amygdala and hippocampus; as we dream, the brain interprets electrical impulses from these emotionally linked areas. Remember: your amygdala is the "fight or flight" part of your brain and the hippocampus stores your memories. One researcher writes, "the amygdala and the hippocampus act synergistically to form long-term memories of significantly emotional events."[20] In other words, the areas of your life that warrant more emotional processing may come out in your dreams.

Dreams are normal and healthy, but if they disrupt your sleep, there are a few factors to examine. Reflecting on your sleep hygiene, discussed in our rituals section, can build self-awareness around the quality of your sleep. Relaxation techniques can help provide more positive dreams and restorative sleep as well.

#CellCare: A sleep tracker is a helpful tool that can inform you how much time you spend in each stage of sleep. It can show differences in body temperature, heart rate, blood pressure, and so on. I use a sleep tracker and always find it fascinating to see the impact of my day's choices on the quality of my sleep.

The length of sleep cycles will vary, depending upon each individual. For example, someone might experience one cycle of all phases in ninety minutes, and in their next full cycle, it might take two hours.

Maybe you'd *love* to get a quality five-stage sleep cycle in—but your body just doesn't seem to want to go there. Or maybe you get eight hours of sleep per night but you still feel tired all day. Let's talk about the *quality* of the sleep you're getting—and how you can make it better.

ALL SLEEP IS NOT CREATED EQUAL

I've said a lot about "quality sleep" in various scientific terms, but on some level, you already know firsthand what it feels like to get a good night's sleep. When you get restful sleep, you start your day feeling energized and rejuvenated; you aren't tired during the day. You're able to function and efficiently perform the tasks you need to. You don't feel the need for caffeine stimulants. You often feel calm, relaxed, and creative, with a clear mind. When you feel this way, it's a good indication you had restful, restorative, quality sleep.

You probably also know firsthand what it means to get poor-quality sleep. You feel tired and lethargic throughout the day; you might feel the need for extra coffee or caffeinated drinks. You tend to feel less focused, irritable, and short-fused. You might notice that you're forgetting things, which would result from not reaching deep stages of your sleep cycle when your memories consolidate. Poor-quality sleep can also result in "emotional constipation," as one of my professors put it. If you don't get to Stage 5, REM sleep, you can't completely process your thoughts, memories, and emotions via your dreams. The result: you get emotionally "backed up."

The recommendations that I'll share in a moment will help improve sleep quality for the average person. However, sleep disorders are real and will require intervention beyond the suggestions in these pages. If you think you may have a sleep disorder, then I recommend a proper sleep evaluation to determine any underlying causes for adequate treatment.

We've already discussed ways to improve sleep by aligning the body's circadian rhythm and sleep–wake homeostasis. However, there's more we can do to experience the rich benefits of restorative rest. First, let's try to avoid sleep sabotage. And second, we can all prioritize intentional sleep hygiene.

Sleep Sabotage

Let's line up the usual suspects of sleep saboteurs:

- ◆ **Caffeine:** Everyone metabolizes caffeine differently; some people will struggle to sleep at night if they have any caffeine after 10:00 a.m. Others can drink coffee into the afternoon without feeling the impact at bedtime. I usually recommend avoiding any caffeine after 2:00 p.m. According to the *Journal of Clinical Sleep Medicine*, caffeine can linger in the body for at least six hours.[21] In some people, caffeine can stick around for up to *twelve* hours.

- ◆ **Alcohol:** While a nightcap may relax you, the alcohol it contains will disrupt your sleep cycle. Although alcohol acts a sedative, making you feel sleepy, it disrupts the quality of your sleep. Even a single glass of wine or beer can wreak havoc on your body while you rest—alcohol disrupts *all* sleep, but it mainly suppresses REM sleep during your first two sleep cycles. As the night progresses, an imbalance is created between REM sleep and deep sleep; this imbalance throws off your sleep duration and quality. Alcohol lingers in the body for two to three hours, so avoiding that drink right before bed can help improve the restorative nature of your sleep.[22] If you do have sleep challenges, cutting out alcohol before bed might be a place to start your ritual focus. Also, if you're leaning on alcohol to help you sleep—unfortunately, that habit will backfire.

♦ **Aerobic activity close to bedtime:** Exercise will increase your heart rate and signal your body to produce adrenaline. These effects can help you wake up in the morning, but if you do a cardio workout in the evening, those effects can disrupt your sleep. So be sure to complete the aerobic exercise at least a few hours before you go to bed. On the other hand, stretching can be an excellent way to help your body relax before sleep.

#**CellCare:** What about sex? In the case of this particular aerobic activity, being physically intimate with your partner can help usher in restful sleep. Sex causes the release of oxytocin, a bonding hormone that can help you feel relaxed. It decreases cortisol, which is the hormone that helps you wake up. An orgasm can also release prolactin, a hormone that causes sleepiness. (Psst: this effect also occurs during masturbation.) There's a reason for the old saying: the bed is for sex and sleep only!

♦ **Late-night snacks:** Eating late at night doesn't give the body adequate time to digest food. When our body is too busy with digestion, blood flow is diverted from the brain to the stomach. As a result, the brain cannot complete the activities it needs to occur in some of the deeper sleep stages, meaning you're more likely to get poor-quality sleep.

♦ **Little cuddlers:** Children and pets in the bed can disrupt sleep—both yours and theirs. It may sound like a cozy idea, but research indicates otherwise.[23]

♦ **Artificial light:** Avoid artificial light before bed, like the blue light from cell phones, iPads, or TVs. These stimulate the brain and trick our bodies into believing it's daylight, which can suppress melatonin production.

#CellCare: Turn off the television. Falling asleep in front of the TV or keeping it on while sleeping is terrible sleep hygiene. Whether you're aware of it or not, your brain is still listening to the sounds of the TV and sensing the flashing lights. You might as well be at a disco party with strobe lights on. The TV disrupts your neuronal pathways, and you won't get quality sleep.

RITUALS FOR SLEEP

A study published in the *Journal of Sleep Research* found an average gap of thirty-nine minutes between the time people go to bed and the time they doze off.[24] That delay may not sound like much, but researchers found that those with a sleep gap of just thirty minutes were three times more likely to have poor sleep quality throughout the rest of the night than people who went to sleep immediately after getting into bed. According to the Centers for Disease Control and Prevention, subpar sleep quality can lead to high blood pressure, heart disease, and weight gain.

Most of us could tighten that sleep gap by improving our sleep hygiene and incorporating some of the sleepy-time rituals I'm about to list. Rituals can benefit your circadian rhythm, which is influenced by your rhythms and habits. For example, when you build a consistent "before bed" routine, you help your body recognize that it's time to produce melatonin and get ready to sleep. That can be a natural gift when your head finally hits the pillow—both for your short-term ability to rest and your long-term health.

Practice Good Sleep Hygiene

If I were your middle-school health teacher instructing you about physical hygiene, I would tell you to do another lap around the field. But since I'm the Wellbeing Doctor and you're a grown adult, I'm going to tell you about sleep hygiene. Sleep hygiene is how you prepare yourself for good, restful sleep. Here's what good sleep hygiene may look like:

♦ Try to keep a consistent sleep schedule, regardless of the day of the week. Even on the weekends, try to go to sleep and wake up around the same time. This consistent pattern helps regulate your circadian rhythm, ensuring you fall asleep more quickly and deeply.

♦ Optimize your bedroom by keeping the temperature cool, blocking any light, and eliminating peripheral noise. A white noise machine can help with this.

♦ If it's within your means, sleep in a comfortable bed. Use a pillow and bedsheets that feel good. You can even use lavender essential oils to calm you and help you sleep.

♦ You might also follow a ritual before bed in the thirty minutes that lead up to sleep time; this routine signals to your body that it's time to rest.

♦ Within three hours of bedtime, avoid alcohol, liquids, caffeine, heavy meals, nicotine, and aerobic exercise.

♦ Review your medications with your physician. One of the most commonly used antidepressants, Prozac, releases serotonin on a continuous basis and can be very stimulating, making it harder to sleep.

Invest in Rest

The most neuroprotective factor of your life is to sleep *well*. In other words, the best thing you can do for your memory, cognition, and mental health is to get good rest. So, if you have concerns about cognitive decline, know that a good night's sleep is essential to maintaining your mental wellbeing.

Therefore, invest the time needed to get sufficient rest. It will give you more years with a greater quality of life in the future! Aim to get between seven to nine hours each night; seven hours is the minimum amount of sleep that will still allow most adults to function optimally.

Napping

Studies have shown that napping can help with the learning process.[25] As a med student, my days were spent buried in books, taking power naps in the library, then waking up and continuing to study. Whether you're a college student, a parent with a young child, or just someone who drags midday, a brief power nap can help your brain rally and re-energize.

The trick with napping is to avoid disrupting your nighttime sleep schedule by napping at inappropriate times. If you nap too late in the day—generally, after 3:00 p.m.—your siesta can backfire. By the time you're ready to go to bed at night, your body and brain won't be prepared to go back to sleep. (That's the sleep–wake homeostasis effect.)

Also, try to keep your nap short, around twenty minutes. You can take a short nap to improve your mood, help you relax, and even enhance your performance and memory without getting into the deeper stages of sleep, which you will find much harder to wake up from. If you nap for too long, you can experience *sleep inertia*, which is when you wake up feeling groggy. Sleep inertia results from sudden awakening during REM sleep, where you still have high levels of melatonin that contribute to sleepiness.

> **#CellCare:** If you're the kind of person who falls asleep as soon as your head hits the pillow, it's an indication that you're overtired and experiencing sleep debt. You may want to try to take a midday power nap. On the other hand, if you go to bed and it takes you twenty minutes or more to fall asleep, you might be experiencing insomnia. Refer back to sleep hygiene for any modifiable actions.

Night Owls

If you're a night owl, work at night, or need to adjust to a different time zone, there are some tricks to simulate conditions conducive for deep sleep. Feel free to make adjustments based on your professional lifestyle and schedule, always in the interest of improving the quality of your sleep.

◆ If you're trying to sleep when it's light out, do your best to simulate nighttime. Use curtains to darken the room.

◆ Use a white noise machine to drown out peripheral sounds. Do your best to minimize or cancel all distractions.

◆ For jet lag, if you arrive at your destination during the day, do your best to avoid falling asleep right away, even if you're tired. Instead, try to stay up until dark. This will help your circadian rhythm realign to the waking hours in your new setting.

If you're a night owl by choice and not because your work demands it, you can train yourself to become more of a morning person. Getting up with the sun and exercising early in the morning can help improve your energy levels and align your circadian rhythm.

Sleep Tracker Apps

Sleep tracking has become popular and is easy to do with smartwatches, rings, and bands. These trackers can be helpful because they can make you aware of your heart rate, HRV, body temperature, and so on. If you don't get good-quality sleep on a particular night, the data from your sleep tracker app can help you to consider the choices you made that day that may have affected your sleep, allowing you to make a more effective plan for tomorrow. Trackers are useful to help you develop a solid sleep routine and identify any potential red flags occurring in your sleep cycle.

Tea Time

Adding tea time to your evening can be a great part of your unwinding routine before sleep. Most people are familiar with chamomile tea as an excellent nighttime option. Chrysanthemum tea is also a great choice: it can clear excessive yang (heat energy) from the liver and calm the nerves. This tea is often recommended in traditional Chinese medicine. Lavender tea is good as well because it can help relax you. Avoid caffeinated teas, such as black or green teas, which are stimulating before bed.

Here are some additional ideas for a sleepy time beverage:

◆ *Chamomile* contains the antioxidant *apigenin* and can help ease anxiety.

◆ *Peppermint* is a good muscle relaxant, therefore helping your body unwind.

◆ *Lemon balm* can increase GABA, contributing to a sedative effect and reducing stress and anxiety.

◆ *Passionflower* can also boost GABA and help with insomnia and anxiety, especially if you feel wired before bed.

◆ *Valerian root* is another GABA booster; although its woody flavor might be an acquired taste, it offers powerful benefits.

◆ *Gotu kola* is a natural remedy for anxiety and insomnia; it also strengthens cognitive function, making it an excellent choice for reducing physical and mental stress.

◆ *Kava* can help relieve stress and anxiety, as well as promote deep sleep without affecting REM sleep.

◆ *Tulsi*—the "queen of herbs" in India—has anti-inflammatory properties and helps manage stress. This tea can help you sleep better if you suffer from indigestion or headaches before bedtime.

#CellCare: Tea is amazing! Tea offers many health benefits, including boosting your immune system, decreasing your blood pressure, reducing stroke risk, aiding with weight loss, preventing bone loss, soothing digestions, and providing beneficial sources of antioxidants. If you're not already a tea drinker, consider this a ritual worth exploring.

Pre-Bed Journaling

Many people have experienced the frustration of having a racing mind when trying to sleep. Pre-bed journaling can help you avoid that, especially if the events of your day stir up strong emotions. The act of journaling can help you unwind before bed, because it activates the left brain's analytical, rational function while allowing the right brain to feel, process, and release the emotions you are expressing. By auditing your day and capturing positive aspects in your journal, you will feel less anxious. By the time you finally doze off, your thoughts will have some order and allow you to achieve some closure.

Brain Dump

A *brain dump* is slightly different from journaling but is also effective in calming you down before sleep. A brain dump is less about articulate emotional processing and more about—well, writing down all the s**t going on inside your mind.

Grab a notebook and jot down what has your brain buzzing. It could be an argument you had with a friend that day, the garbage you read on Twitter, or social issues that need to be solved. Once you write them down, you know you can return to them in the morning and allow yourself to forget them while falling asleep.

Plan for Tomorrow

Whether putting your clothes out for work, packing your bag for the gym, preparing your lunch, or writing a to-do list, getting organized for the following day can ease your mind before bed. There's science behind this: a cognitive process called *proactive coping* can alleviate stress through advanced preparation.[26] Additionally, planning reduces cognitive overload since the human brain can only process a limited amount of information at a time. We can all agree that uncertainty causes us to feel powerless, which leads to stress. However, by preparing in advance, you can anticipate and make plans to deal with potential stress. Make a plan, any plan.

Sacred Soak

Water can be therapeutic and soothe your mind. If you're feeling wound up, try taking a warm shower or a bath with essential oils. Rose, jasmine, and lavender can reduce stress and relieve negative emotions. The experience can calm the nervous system, decreasing anxiety and stress.

You get this mood boost because of the effect of the water's temperature. When your body temperature rises in a warm bath, the subsequent relaxing of your body cues your parasympathetic nervous system to start releasing serotonin and dopamine, your feel-good hormones. Additionally, the warm water helps regulate your body temperature, which can promote better sleep; in fact, studies show that taking a bath one to two hours before bedtime can help you fall asleep faster.[27]

Pre-Bed Stretch

The evening is the perfect time to get on the floor with your child or pet and stretch out your entire body. The benefits of stretching include stress relief, enhanced mood, improved mobility, improved circulation, and reduced body pain. Overall, stretching can relieve stress from the day and signal the relaxation process for sleep. Give the following stretches a try: legs up the wall, butterfly (while sitting, put your feet together and gently flutter your knees), head rolls, and spinal twist.

Evening Playlist

Making an evening playlist with soothing sounds will signal to your brain that it's time to sleep. Some people prefer classical music; others prefer relaxing ambient sounds, like waves; you could even include ancestral sounds, like didgeridoos or a hand pan. Relaxing music can help you cope with stress and sleep better by slowing your breathing, lowering your heart rate and decreasing your blood pressure. Use your playlist while brushing your teeth or washing your face to incorporate the sound experience into your bedtime ritual. Here are a few more tips to create your first bedtime playlist: look for music with slow-moving tones, use it consistently every night, and adjust as needed.

Abhyanga

Abhyanga is an Ayurvedic massage using warm oil to smooth the skin, cleanse the lymphatic system, and soothe the nervous system; it is highly effective in relaxing the body. This loving ritual is traditionally offered in the mornings. Still, it can also be a beautiful way to nourish and ground yourself in the evening, relieving any excess tension from your busy day. Pair it with your evening bath by offering it to yourself before or after your soak in the tub. Use slow, long, heavy strokes and a calming herbal-infused body oil to support your ultimate sleep goals.

Acupressure Behind the Ear

Located behind the ear is an acupressure point called *anmian*, which translates to "peaceful sleep" and is used to treat insomnia.

It's found between the ear and the base of the skull, where there's a slight depression next to a bone called the mastoid process. Place your finger on this depression and apply pressure in a circular motion to massage it. After circling a hundred times, you should feel more relaxed and ready to rest.

Yoga Nidra

This is a form of guided meditation, a method of *pratyahara* (withdrawal of the senses) that allows you to scan the body and tap into a state of relaxed consciousness as the mind settles into a place between wakefulness and sleep.

When you start yoga nidra, your brain is generally in an active state of beta waves, a natural transitional experience as you slow down and press pause on your day. The meditative practice then takes you deeper into an alpha state, the brain wave frequency that links conscious thought with the subconscious mind.

In the alpha state, serotonin is released, which helps you reach a transformational experience of inner calm. From this place, fluctuations in your mind start to decrease, and you begin to feel more at ease. Finally, the body moves into stillness, and a deep feeling of tranquility and relaxation occurs. As you move deeper into the practice, the brain will begin to emit delta waves, mimicking what happens when we enter a night of deep, restful sleep. The difference between deep sleep and yoga nidra is staying awake during this final phase.

The regular practice of yoga nidra can counteract the effects of stress and hyperactivity of the brain's frontal cortex, putting us in a restorative state. People who have sleep issues often experience a noticeable improvement in their sleep when starting a yoga nidra ritual.

Power Down

As discussed earlier, the blue light from electronics has a wavelength similar to sunlight, disrupting your circadian rhythms and natural ability to fall asleep. Therefore, devices should be shut down thirty minutes before bedtime, and notifications should be turned off. This ritual will be hard, but if you are experiencing any difficulty with quality sleep, it will also be one of the most effective. Start by putting a curfew on your electronics, adding a book by your bedside, and investing in some blue-light blocking glasses.

SLEEP:
THAT GOLDEN CHAIN

The English dramatist Thomas Dekker once wrote, "Sleep is that golden chain that ties health and our bodies together." Although he penned those words more than four hundred years ago, his observation was accurate—sleep is an essential link between our bodies and our physical and mental wellbeing.

It can be easy to deprioritize sleep in favor of other, more exciting or seemingly more important activities, like working late or staying up with friends. Perhaps we underestimate the value of sleep since we're unconscious while it happens! However, tremendously important biological processes only occur when we allow our bodies to rest deeply. These processes are critical for our cognitive longevity and long-term health. Sleep makes us better, kinder, more sociable, and happier human beings. It truly is a golden chain that ties our bodies to health and wellbeing.

Reflect on Your #CellCare

Using these guiding questions, take a moment to build self-awareness and reflect on the quality of sleep in your life:

- Do you have trouble falling asleep or staying asleep, or do you wake in the night?

- Do you feel refreshed when you wake in the morning?

- Do you experience daytime sleepiness and the need for naps?

- Do you feel irritable and short-fused from disrupted sleep?

- Do you have a regular sleep–wake rhythm?

DESIGN YOUR WELLBEING

In the space below, note your thoughts about your current sleep hygiene. Then, name a ritual you may want to incorporate into your life to improve your overall sleep and note how often you would like to do it.

7

ELIMINATING HIDDEN TOXINS

"Maintaining one's health in today's toxic rich environment requires proper rest, hydration, an abundant intake of nutrients, and regular internal cleansing practices."

~ GARY HOPKINS, AUTHOR OF THE MASTER WITHIN

BREE CAME TO MY OFFICE TO DISCUSS HER DIFFICULTLY getting pregnant. She very much wanted to become a mom but wasn't ready to go down the road of fertility treatments. She hoped there might be something else she could do to work on her health to naturally increase her fertility, and she asked for my help.

We talked through several areas of her lifestyle, but one topic quickly emerged as a noteworthy hindrance: her exposure to environmental factors. I gave Bree a questionnaire that asked about her food intake, living environment, travel, and personal care. That last item got her attention. Personal care products were a major fixture in Bree's life. One of her favorite outings was a trip to Sephora to get all the latest beauty products—everything from lipsticks to foundations to new hair products. She also loved going to the hair salon to get a professional blowout and updated coloring. Bree wasn't conscious of what ingredients might be in any of these products; mainly, she chose products based on whether they would enhance her beauty.

The problem was those products were also likely affecting her fertility and overall wellbeing. Unless her products had been carefully curated for their ingredients, I knew that years of heavy beauty product use most likely meant that Bree had absorbed many chemicals. However, I was most concerned about her exposure to endocrine disrupters, which can significantly impact hormone production, including reproductive hormones for fertility.

I asked Bree to bring in all her beauty products for the next appointment. She did—piles of them. My desk was loaded with makeup, shampoo, conditioner, body lotion, sunblock, styling products, perfume, and even toothpaste. She brought in *every* product that she put on her body. Then, one by one, we started reading the labels. The process led to an extensive discussion about key ingredients to watch out for, the impact those ingredients could have on her cellular health, and ways Bree could begin to clean up this area of her life.

It didn't happen overnight. Bree had invested a lot of money into many of these products, and she didn't want to throw them out, nor was she prepared to stop wearing makeup or styling her hair. But over the next year, every time she ran out of one of her products, Bree made a point of replacing it with something that had cleaner ingredients. Rather than looking for brands that were well marketed or trendy, she looked for brands with a reputation for natural clean ingredients.

Of course, we worked on other areas of her life—Bree also changed her exercise, diet, emotional self-care, and sleep habits. Remember that an integrative lifestyle involves a whole-body approach, respecting that everything in our body is closely intertwined. However, to eliminate any potential factors affecting her hormones and fertility, Bree's most significant lifestyle change targeted the environmental toxins in her life.

Bree arrived for an appointment about a year later with some happy news: she was thirteen weeks pregnant! Bree had changed her body's ability to get pregnant mainly through alterations in her daily routines, without ever taking fertility treatment. After making purposeful lifestyle changes, Bree is now the mother of a beautiful baby girl.

Here's the truth: environmental toxins are all around us. Without an intentional effort to limit them, you will be exposed to them constantly. Moreover, toxins that accumulate over time have a consistent, adverse effect on your body. However, in making an effort to remove toxic elements in your environment, you can fortify your cells, optimize your body's functions, and transform your wellbeing.

WHERE ARE THE WARNING LABELS?

When I start talking with my patients about environmental toxins, many are surprised by how widespread they are. How can so many industries get away with selling products that damage our health? I recently hosted a toxic beauty panel, and someone asked, "If a product is on store shelves, can't I assume it's passed safety standards required by the FDA?" Unfortunately, it's not that simple.

Just because a product is on the shelf in a store does not necessarily mean it's gone through exceptional approval. For instance, the FDA *regulates* cosmetics but does not have the legal authority to *approve* them in the same way they would approve a medication. This means they check to see if a product is poisonous, misbranded, or has color additives—but that's as far as they may go. Other products fall entirely outside their jurisdiction, like cleaning products, home renovation products, or pet-related products such as cat litter. These are items that people buy and use every day, but many are not regulated.

That means the responsibility to 'fess up about potentially harmful ingredients is on the companies themselves. Thankfully, in recent years, there's been consumer pressure on companies to be more transparent about the ingredients in their products. You might have seen notices on certain products like "contains no parabens" or "BPA-free." Companies often market themselves as having strong commitments to consumer safety.

But here's a scary truth: one of the leading environmental toxins, *endocrine disrupters,* are found nearly everywhere: in personal care products, children's toys, anything plastic, detergents, food packaging, pharmaceuticals, and in many, many other products. These endocrine disrupters impact our entire endocrine system, and their effect is enormous. *But regulators have yet to determine what a safe level is.* No wonder my patient Bree had no idea her beauty products might be having such a detrimental effect on her health.

Companies are not obligated to inform you of these incredibly commonplace toxins and can include any amount in their products and packaging. There are also ways to get around even the loose regulations imposed by the FDA. For instance, the word "perfume" (parfum) leads to an easy loophole. Perfumes are incredibly bad for our bodies—they contain allergens,[1] endocrine disrupters,[2] asthma triggers,[3] neurotoxins,[4] and carcinogens[5]—which means that anything scented may contain toxins. However, there's no defined list of what ingredients fall under the category of "perfume." As a result, companies can list an ingredient that most consumers won't recognize or make a new variation with a new name—like "fragrance"—and sell a new product containing toxic ingredients.

> #**CellCare:** The organization Environmental Work-
> ing Group (EWG) has a website that allows you to
> enter nearly any household or beauty product to see
> its level of toxicity. Moreover, it provides toxicity
> scores for each ingredient listed in the product, indi-
> cating whether it is harmful or not. It's a great tool!
> You can find it at: www.ewg.org. In addition, you can
> check out EWG Skin Deep to find out what toxins are
> in your personal care products, and EWG Tap Water
> Database to view toxins in your water.

As of 2020, there were *167 million* chemicals registered with the American Chemical Society, but less than *one percent* of those chemicals were tested for toxicity. And—more bad news—the less-than-one percent of chemicals tested were determined to be toxic enough to disrupt essentially every cellular process in the body. Given the widespread nature of these environmental toxins and the current lax industry standards for regulation, it's the consumer's responsibility to educate themselves and look out for them. If you think that's a drag—I agree with you.

It might be tempting to conclude that all this talk about toxins is overblown. And taking a complete inventory of all your environmental toxins probably sounds time consuming, inconvenient, and expensive—not to mention scary. So, is it worth trying to decontaminate your life of toxins?

Perhaps if I share just a little of what toxins do to your body, you can decide if it's worth your #CellCare.

HOW TOXINS IMPACT OUR BODIES

There are at least eight ways toxins interfere with our bodies at a cellular level. Although these changes are largely invisible to the eye, we feel their short and long-term effects.

1. Damage DNA and Modify Gene Expression

As discussed in Chapter Three, every one of your cells contains DNA, and this DNA suffers one of the worst attacks from toxins. Some toxins are known as genotoxins because they directly impact your genetic code.[6] That can cause damage to your DNA and chromosomes, ultimately leading to diverse diseases, including cancer.[7]

In Chapter Two, I explained the concept of *epigenetics*. Remember, that's the process of some genes being "on" or "off" related to environmental influences. Some of those genes are permanently turned on, like the ones that determine your height, hair color, and eye color. Other, less visible genes will also always be turned on, like those that determine your metabolism, digestive health, and sleep–wake cycle.

Other genes along this chain are turned off—in other words, they are inactive, provided your DNA remains healthy. For instance, you might have a genetic variant linked to heart disease. This gene might remain turned off if you can maintain a healthy lifestyle and give your body what it needs to thrive. Just because you possess that gene does not necessarily mean you will experience a heart attack or chronic heart disease. The gene is there, but it can remain turned off, and you'd never be bothered by it.

However, your cellular health can be compromised when you introduce toxins into your system. Everything you are exposed to—from the nutrients (or lack thereof) you get from your diet to the environmental exposures you experience—impacts the health of your DNA. If you provide your body with ingredients it needs to produce healthy cells, then as they replicate, they will be normal functioning cells. However, if your body is exposed to an abundance of harmful toxins, the replicated cells are likely to be unhealthy. Those unhealthy cells will almost always have a ripple effect. One of the most common ripple effects of damaged DNA is *dysplasia*, which is the abnormal growth of cells that can ultimately lead to cancer.

Toxins are a major contributing factor impacting your cellular health, and specifically, the healthy production of DNA. Therefore, avoiding them is one of the best ways you can optimize the health of your cells, thereby minimizing contributing factors to chronic illness.

2. Damage Cell Signals

One of the incredible ways your body regulates and initiates all the different processes that constantly occur inside you happens via cellular communication. For instance, imagine eating a piece of cake and giving your body a major dose of glucose. Inside your body, your cells pass along that message—"Glucose!"—to the pancreas via the cell membranes. The cell membranes are its communication center— think of a healthy cell membrane as equivalent to a robust, four-bar cell signal (pun intended). With healthy cell membranes and strong communication signals between cells, the message of "Glucose!" reaches the cells of the pancreas, and the pancreas begins producing insulin, therefore helping the body metabolize the glucose.

But imagine that those cell signals get damaged. Suddenly, the cells' ability to communicate key messages to each other is compromised, in the same way that your ability to call your friend would be compromised if you lost cell service. With a damaged cell membrane, that glucose message isn't getting through. As a result, your body can't metabolize sugar properly, and you end up with high blood sugar. That can further compromise your body's healthy functioning.

Toxins cause damage to those cell membranes, which means they hinder the crucial communication that needs to occur among your cells for so many of your essential body functions.

3. Interfere with Hormone Production

Now, if your cells can't communicate effectively with one another, you can bet that a host of problems will result. One of the biggest?

ELIMINATING HIDDEN TOXINS

Toxins can interfere with your hormone production. As discussed in Bree's story, an enormous class of environmental toxins called endocrine disrupters explicitly targets your hormones. We'll discuss these endocrine disrupters more later in this chapter—but first, let's consider their effect on the body.

Here are just a few of the hormones that toxins can interfere with:

♦ **Serotonin:** The hormone that helps you feel happy.

♦ **Estrogen and progesterone:** Hormones that influence a woman's fertility.

♦ **Testosterone:** A hormone that boosts confidence and impacts virility in a man.

♦ **Oxytocin:** A hormone that helps you build close, loving relationships.

♦ **Melatonin:** The hormone that enables you to sleep well.

In other words: healthy hormone production is not something you want to mess with. But that's precisely what toxins do. Their interference with your hormone production can cause imbalances, leading to issues like depression, infertility, anxiety, and more. That's possibly why eliminating the beauty products full of endocrine disrupters made a difference in Bree's fertility journey. Those disrupters were inhibiting her body's cellular messaging system, meaning there was an imbalanced production of hormones. When she removed those toxins, her cellular health improved, those cells could communicate critical messages, and her body could produce the hormones it needed to conceive.

4. Interfere with Enzymatic Processes

Equally as important to your body's wellbeing are your enzymatic processes, or your body's chemical reactions. An enzyme is a type of protein found in a cell. It is the catalyst that regulates the rate of your body's chemical reactions. For instance, several organs produce digestive enzymes, like the salivary glands, the pancreas, and the small intestine. It is these enzymes that help break down the food you eat, but if they don't work well, those chemical reactions will not take place as efficiently as they should. As a result, you digest your food more slowly, less effectively, and with more discomfort, and you might have problems absorbing nutrients.

What are these enzymatic processes responsible for? *Every physiologic function in the body.* They're responsible for making your energy. They affect the production of your red blood cells, which impacts your oxygen levels. They affect the production of your white blood cells, which impacts your immune system. They affect your neurotransmitters, which influence communication in your brain. When toxins damage your enzymatic processes, they damage everything. So ultimately, if you want to keep those catalysts functional, eliminating environmental toxins is a priority.

5. Impact Your Body's Ability to Remove Toxins

As we're about to discuss in the next section of this chapter, your body has an amazing ability to remove toxins. Six major body systems work together to remove all the gross stuff we're exposed to. You can think of these body systems as a top-notch team of house cleaners. They're ready to go head to head with the grime and muck in your body and clean it out.

However, many toxins prevent your body from effectively removing them. Imagine that your team of Merry Maids® suddenly finds itself face to face with an enormous mess—like a nuclear waste spill or something on the level of the food poisoning scene from the movie *Bridesmaids*. The level of those toxins will paralyze your body's ability to deal with them effectively. This is beyond your body's cleaning team scope!

Unfortunately, when your body's toxin-removal systems are compromised, the toxins have very little holding them back from causing more widespread damage. The harmful effects of toxins we just discussed will be compounded because the protective systems cannot function properly to stop them. Picture each of your house cleaners suddenly breaking an ankle: they're simply no longer able to carry out their job. Even if just one or two of your body systems suffers a broken ankle, you can imagine the strain that would put on the other toxin-removal systems. As they try to make up for the missing helpers, those other systems can more easily become overwhelmed.

6. Increase Your Rate of Aging

If toxins are battering away at your DNA, it stands to reason that your body will start to show the visible effects of those compromised cells. You can think about this in terms of the chassis of a car. I spent many years living on the east coast, where there were often terrible snowstorms in the winter months. After every snowstorm, the roads were covered with salt to help speed up the melting of the ice. However, as cars drove over the streets, that salt collected in the wheel wells and on the undercarriage of the chassis. Over time, that salt corroded the metal, leaving holes and rust patches. If I didn't make a point of cleaning those toxins off my car, I knew my car would age more rapidly than it would otherwise.

The same thing happens to your body when it encounters toxins like PAHs (polycyclic aromatic hydrocarbons), which are generated from cooking, smoking, or vehicle exhaust combustion.[8] You may not be able to avoid road or city pollution, but you can limit your exposure to PAHs by ensuring that you cook in a well-ventilated area and avoid smoking. Imagine that those toxins are coating your cells with a layer of grime—like road salt covering a car's undercarriage. As a result, they lead to the degeneration of your DNA, increasing your aging rate. In other words, exposure to toxins will make you look older.

7. Displace Needed Nutrients

Finally, toxins also displace other necessary minerals and nutrients. For example, calcium is an essential nutrient for bone health. Typically, you absorb quite a bit of calcium from your food, but toxins can prevent that healthy absorption from occurring. Furthermore, the toxins take the place of calcium. So rather than your body flushing toxins from your system and absorbing the calcium, it's the calcium that gets flushed and the toxins that get absorbed. The result is bone loss.

When you consider all the ways that toxins cause harm to your body, the conclusion seems obvious: we can do a lot better. For example, we can remove many of the environmental toxins we're currently exposed to and prioritize keeping our toxin-removal systems in good health.

Speaking of those toxin-removal heroes, let's take a break from the doom and gloom and talk about the incredible systems in your body that clean us up from the inside out.

HOW THE BODY REMOVES TOXINS

The good news is our cells have a remarkable ability to self-clean and address chemical damage. There are six systems in the body that naturally remove toxins, and trust me—you need every one of them.

- ◆ **Skin:** Your skin is the largest organ in your body. It protects you from external toxins, like bacteria and UV radiation. Furthermore, your body eliminates heavy metals and other toxic chemicals when you sweat.[9] (Note: If you don't sweat regularly via exercise or sauna, make that a ritual!)

- ◆ **Kidneys:** Part of your *genitourinary* system, the kidneys are responsible for purifying the blood by filtering toxic chemicals out of the blood and excreting them into your urine. Then, they can be flushed from your body. Given the kidneys' responsibility for cleaning up your blood, it's no surprise that people with high blood pressure also have kidney issues. You can support your kidneys' health by reducing sodium in your diet, staying well hydrated, and eating whole, fresh foods with lots of fiber.[10]

- **Digestive System:** Throughout your digestive process, toxins may enter your bloodstream through your food or drink. If your gut is in check and the cells lining it are strong and healthy, then those toxins will be removed. However, as discussed in Chapter Four, with an unhealthy gut lining, the toxins can enter the bloodstream and go to other parts of your body. A high-fiber diet can help toxins "latch on," ensuring that they hitch a ride out of your body rather than being absorbed into your body.

- **Liver:** The liver—one of your toxin-removal all-stars—is responsible for deactivating and removing the toxic substances you get from medication, excess hormones, food additives, and more. The liver takes toxic waste out of your blood and transforms the waste into something that can be excreted via your intestines or kidneys (i.e., your stool or urine). In that way, it's like the team captain of the toxin-removal squad: it does its thing, then passes the ball to either the kidneys or digestive tract so that they can finish the job. Even though your liver is a toxin-removal all-star, your lifestyle habits can severely affect your liver's healthy functioning. Drinking, smoking, taking too much medication, having poor nutrition, not getting enough sleep—all of these habits overburden your liver, impeding its ability to clean your body's blood. That's why a heavy drinker will have a much harder time removing toxins like cancer-causing agents and endocrine disrupters. This is true even if you have quit drinking, unfortunately. A history of heavy alcohol consumption or medication use can cause

DNA damage, and that DNA damage is the precursor to several diseases, including cancer. Alcohol doesn't just damage liver cells; it damages all cells.

♦ **Respiratory System:** Your lungs and bronchi are critical players in your body's toxin-removal systems. When you inhale, you breathe in a combination of oxygen and nitrogen. Your lungs filter out the oxygen and send it into the bloodstream; then, they send carbon dioxide—a waste product—out of your body via your exhale. When you don't have efficient breathing mechanisms, your body can't remove toxins as effectively. Therefore, learning to breathe well is a considerable component of helping your body heal. With impaired breathing, the body is put at a severe disadvantage to remove toxins from the body, making recovery a much slower process.

♦ **Lymphatic System:** The lymphatic system is another top defender against toxins and has locations throughout the body: in the lymph nodes, the spleen, the sinuses, and so on. These locales are all connected via the lymphatic system, which runs alongside the vascular system: your arteries carry blood from the heart to your organs; veins carry the blood away from your organs, and the lymphatic system carries toxins away. This is one reason you might notice swollen lymph nodes when you're sick: the extra toxins in your body are collecting in the tissue of your lymph nodes, where cells known as macrophages gobble them up to get rid of them. The lymphatic system is fundamental in the detoxification pathway. You can boost the lymphatic system with massage, dry brushing, exercise, limiting processed foods, drinking plenty of water, and of course, eating your fruits and vegetables.

One area of the body that's decidedly *unhelpful* at removing toxins is your fat. Although it's healthy to have some body fat (for men, a healthy range of body fat is 8 to 19 percent; for women, 21 to 33 percent), too much body fat can tax your body in many ways. There are several well-known drawbacks of having surplus body fat, but a less familiar fact is that surplus body fat serves as toxin storage. So, while the body systems on your toxin-removal team are trying to get toxins *out* of your system, your fat happily holds onto them, providing toxins with a plush, comfortable seating area. Take that as one more reason to work up a sweat!

Consider Your Toxic Burden

How do you know if toxins are harming your body? Start by taking a look at how your body is functioning. These common symptoms can signify that your body is overloaded with toxins:

- ◆ Brain fog

- ◆ Sleep problems

- ◆ Mood issues

- ◆ Anxiety

- ◆ Fatigue

- Muscle aches

- Joint pain

- Headaches

- Bloating and flatulence

- Weight changes

- Fluid retention

- Skin rashes

These symptoms are your body's way of telling you that your toxin-removal pathways are overburdened. Therefore, your body needs your help to get those systems back on track. If you experience many of the listed symptoms, the best thing you can do for your body is to work on alleviating your exposure to environmental toxins and make sure you're giving your toxin-removal systems the ingredients they need to thrive.

If you recognize a need to detox, you might conclude that you should detox diet—but I would discourage that. There's no shortage of trendy detox diets out there: some people go on a juice cleanse; others might get enemas; some people might take a break from alcohol—fully intending to resume their drinking habits down the road. However, many of these heavily restrictive cleanses can cause more stress to your body than benefits. A juice cleanse, for instance, will give your digestion a rest, but it may deprive your body of other nutrients it needs. It's also common for people to use detox diets as a crutch—for instance, you go on vacation for a week and binge on alcohol and rich food, telling yourself you'll do a detox once you're home. However, when you've been in "Fat Tuesday" mode, then abruptly shift to super clean eating, the body will struggle to adjust. That can lead people to conclude that "eating healthy" just isn't working for them. One patient told me once, "My bowels work better when I drink." Actually, she simply hadn't given her body a chance to adjust to cleaner living. In all fairness, alcohol can increase gut motility (movement), but you don't get ideal stools; you can also damage your digestive tract. Changing your lifestyle slowly, steadily, and consistently will benefit you in the long run.

> **#CellCare:** "I'm usually bloated. But that's normal, right?" "I'm always constipated. I think that's pretty typical." "I have brain fog again." I hear these comments from people often who have convinced themselves that these symptoms are normal. They're not normal! There's something you can do to heal your body in these areas. Consider your toxicity exposure—there's a good chance some of these symptoms are related to environmental toxins. Work on cutting out areas of toxins and support your body's toxin-removal systems by incorporating some of this chapter's rituals.

Your body will be much more effective at removing toxins if you simply focus on giving its natural toxin-removal systems the nutrients they need to function well. Remember: your body is made to do this. It has systems entirely devoted to removing toxins! When detoxifying, it's just as important to focus on appropriate replacement and replenishment as it is to focus on removing. Thoughtfully incorporate a few new rituals into your life to help your body sustain its toxin removal efficacy for the long term.

CHIEF OFFENDERS

Toxins are not just manmade chemicals; they also include bacteria, viruses, parasites, allergens, and even medications—basically, anything that is harmful to your body. Speaking of removal, it's high time we identified some of the key culprits wreaking havoc on your body. Let's start with our top offender.

Endocrine Disrupting Chemicals (EDC)

This toxic culprit is found in nearly everything. On the team of EDCs, there are several villainous players:

- ◆ **Parabens** are found in many beauty and skincare products. Watch for ingredients where paraben is part of the name; often, the ingredients will look like "sodium butylparaben" or "methylparaben." These toxins interfere with normal hormone production and can negatively impact reproduction and fertility in anyone.

- ◆ **Phthalates** make plastic more flexible and durable, but they can lead to health issues. And unfortunately, they're found nearly everywhere—think of everything you touch every day made from plastic! Phthalates are found in pharmaceuticals, children's toys, detergent, food packaging, soaps, shampoos, and many personal care products, such as aftershave, lotion, soap, shampoos, perfumes, hair spray, nail polish, and so on.

♦ **Triclosan** is often found in antibacterial soaps, lotions, some cosmetics, many body washes, and toothpaste.

♦ **BPA** is a harmful chemical used in many plastics like Tupperware and plastic water bottles linked to adverse health effects such as early pregnancy loss and placental diseases. Additionally, BPA acts as a potent oxidant that can alter cell growth, activating inflammatory cytokines and triggering EGFR/KRAS signaling factors associated with the development of lung cancer.[11] Consumers have largely caught on to the dangers of BPA, so you'll notice advertising touting a product as "BPA free." However, even BPA-free plastic is full of potentially harmful chemicals and poses a threat to the environment.[12]

Collectively, this vile group of EDCs has been shown to interact with a wide variety of our cell membrane receptors (remember: that's how our cells communicate with each other). They also hit our neurotransmitters, which impact our production of the hormones serotonin and dopamine (our "happy" hormones) and norepinephrine (which provides energy to the body), among others.[13] They affect our entire endocrine system (i.e., *all* of our hormones) and our neurotransmitters (i.e., our cognition). And let me repeat my doomsday warning from earlier: researchers *have yet to determine what a safe level is.*

EFFECTS OF
ENDOCRINE-DISRUPTING CHEMICALS

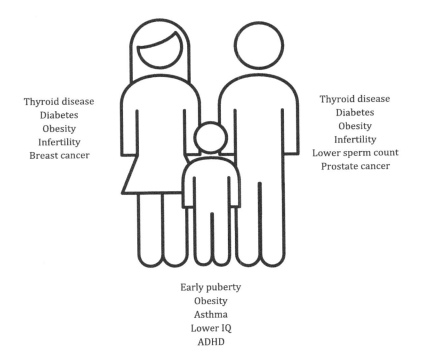

Thyroid disease
Diabetes
Obesity
Infertility
Breast cancer

Thyroid disease
Diabetes
Obesity
Infertility
Lower sperm count
Prostate cancer

Early puberty
Obesity
Asthma
Lower IQ
ADHD

What does it look like when EDCs impact your body? In children, EDC toxins are linked to early puberty, asthma, obesity, hyperactivity, ADHD, and lower IQ levels—just to name a few. Among women, EDC toxins have been linked to thyroid problems, breast cancer, diabetes, obesity, and infertility. Many of these same health issues impact men—plus prostate cancer and low sperm count. People don't often think about using plastic Tupperware, applying face cream, or giving their child a rubber ducky in the bath—but frankly, these everyday items can conspire to cause serious health issues to our loved ones and us.

261

#CellCare: Rather than using plastic containers to store your food, I recommend using glass, metal, or bamboo containers. In the case of plastic lids, avoid letting the food touch the plastic, and wash the plastic lids by hand. Heat from the dishwasher—even on the top shelf—breaks down plastic over time, posing a health risk.

Medications

You might be surprised to see medications on this list of chief offenders. But think about the last pharmaceutical TV ad you heard—there's usually a long list of side effects listed at the end, either in tiny fine print or spoken very fast. Most people assume that if a doctor prescribes medication, it must be good for them. However, traditional medical systems focus on symptom alleviation—which medications are good for. What medications can't do, though, is reverse disease.

Medications can become toxic with overuse or when combined poorly with other medications. Sometimes, they can end up causing harm in one area while they're helping another. For example, antacid medications are commonly prescribed for acid reflux. However, taking these medications for years can impair kidney function and cause bone fractures. Birth control pills can also be a major culprit; when taken for many years, they can lead to vitamin deficiencies in B12, B6, vitamin C, magnesium, and zinc—all vital to your health.

Does that mean you shouldn't take medication at all? No; there are certainly times when medicine is necessary and appropriate.

Medications, however, are like band-aids: they may temporarily alleviate symptoms, but they won't get down to the root cause of why you were experiencing those symptoms in the first place. Sometimes, you simply need that symptom alleviation. For example, if you have a migraine, take a pain killer and alleviate that symptom—but don't stop there. Instead, do your best to figure out why those migraines are happening in the first place. Understanding your body's functioning will help you take care of it holistically.

Other Offenders

There are many other categories of toxins to be aware of including: *chemical* (the manmade kind), *biologic* (like viruses, bacteria, parasites), *radiation* (such as X-rays and UV rays), *physical* (like coal dust, asbestos, gases, etc.), and *behavioral* (a slight misnomer, "behavioral" toxicity refers to therapeutic levels of medications, which can have potentially damaging side effects). Keeping that in mind, here are a few other toxins to avoid:

◆ **Anti-nutrients** are dietary toxins that include high-fructose corn syrups, caffeine, trans fats, alcohol, processed foods, and GMOs, among others. (Remember: GMO means "genetically modified organisms," which are unnatural.) Although many brands have started noting that their foods are GMO-free, it's worth noting that GMOs are still present in upwards of 75 percent of processed foods on supermarket shelves—yikes.

263

♦ **Internal metabolic toxins**—like bile, stool, urine, carbon dioxide, nitrogen, free radicals, chemicals, and so on—are our body's breakdown products. These toxins are made from whatever we put into our body, and as discussed, our body has systems in place to get them out—provided we help keep those systems healthy.

♦ **Heavy metals**—not the Black Sabbath kind—are toxins that show up in our blood. Some of the harmful heavy metals I see most often in my patients' blood tests include mercury, arsenic, lead, cadmium, aluminum, and tin. Where do these come from? Mercury often sneaks into our bodies via seafood—especially if you eat a lot of it. Our water supply can contain arsenic and lead, and aluminum is an active ingredient in many deodorants. Heavy metals are also in many beauty products and certain toothpastes.

♦ **Allergens** are a type of toxin that will also cramp your style: mold, dust, pollen, certain foods, and pet dander are the most common offenders. Try to improve your indoor air quality by reducing humidity, which reduces dust mites and mold growth. Also, keeping your home clean and uncluttered will help. (More on that in our next chapter!) Avoid wall-to-wall carpet if possible, which can trap many allergens in its fibers. Finally, if you allow your pets to sleep on your bed, make sure you're washing your sheets weekly.

♦ **Infectious organisms** are our most familiar toxic culprit: we know these make us sick. Infectious organisms include bacteria, viruses, parasites, fungus, and protozoa. Keep in mind we can pick these up anywhere, especially when traveling.

♦ **Obesogens** are chemicals that alter lipid homeostasis (fat cell balance). Over time, they increase fat cells, negatively affect metabolism, and impact the gut microbiome. These compounds are found in everyday products, including personal care products, cookware, toys, food containers, medical supplies, and cleaning agents. BPA, phthalates, atrazine (herbicides), organotins (pesticides), and PFOA (found in nonstick cookware and microwaveable food items) are all examples of common obesogens.

♦ **Fluoride** is probably the sneakiest culprit. Yes: fluoride makes the list. This ingredient is added to our water and toothpaste (not to mention those gooey dentist trays) for our dental health. However, fluoride likes to deposit and concentrate in certain areas. One of its favorite spots to set up camp is in our pineal gland, the part of our brain responsible for making the melatonin that helps us sleep. Some studies have found that long-term fluoride exposure can displace the normal production of melatonin, ultimately affecting sleep.[14] Additionally, fluoride has been linked to a number of health problems in the categories of cardiovascular, reproductive, neurologic, joint, and skin issues.[15] Here's the thing: fluoride already naturally occurs in water, soil, and food. It's *synthetically* added to toothpaste, mouthwashes, and most drinking water. You're likely getting more than enough fluoride already, so avoid it where you can.

♦ **Environmental chemicals**, like pesticides, herbicides, fungicides, insecticides (basically anything lawn-related), cleaning products, household products, and—once again—beauty products, comprise another key culprit. You can limit these by seeking out natural lawn maintenance care and natural cleaners.

> **#CellCare:** Pesticides are especially harmful for the body, and they have both short term and long term effects; children are the most susceptible to them. Short-term effects might be dizziness, diarrhea, rashes, and nausea. Even if you don't experience these short-term symptoms, pesticides can accumulate in your body and lead to some scary long-term consequences. Pesticides are linked to many types of cancers, such as breast,[16] brain,[17] prostate,[18] and leukemia/lymphoma.[19] Unfortunately, many pesticides end up in our water supply. You can do your best to reduce pesticide absorption by eating organic foods and filtering your water.

RITUALS FOR WELLBEING

Now for the good news. There are many purposeful rituals you can incorporate into the rhythms of your life to aid your body's natural ability to purge toxins. These rituals can help you clean up your toxic exposure and start to flush accumulated toxins in your body. Not all damage from toxins is permanent—these intentional practices can help revitalize your cells.

Ayurvedic Rituals

These ancient Ayurvedic rituals can help your body naturally detox:

◆ **Jiwah Prakshalan (tongue scraping):** Before you brush your teeth, scrape your tongue using a metal U-shaped tongue scraper tool. (You can find one of these by looking up "tongue scraper" on Amazon or find one at Whole Foods). Lots of bacteria accumulate in your mouth, which can change its level of acidity, contributing to plaque buildup and eventually gum disease. Tongue scraping helps remove many of those toxins before they ever manage to work their way into the rest of your body. Consider tongue scraping as part of your oral hygiene ritual. The order will vary from expert to expert, but my suggestion is to tongue scrape, floss, brush, mouthwash twice a day—morning and night. As you begin including tongue scraping into your ritual, you will know when you have been doing an excellent job based upon the amount of gunk being scraped off; after doing it consistently for a while, you'll start to see less and less.

◆ **Gharsana (the Ayurvedic version of dry brushing)** can help your lymphatic system. A dry brush looks like a loofah on a handle. Using the dry brush, start at the ankles and move toward the heart; brush the front of both legs, then the back; move to the arms, bringing the brush from distal to proximal; and go in clockwise circular motions over the abdomen. The brushing stimulates lymphatic drainage and increases blood circulation, aiding your body's toxin-removal process. Some people claim dry brushing also helps remove cellulite as a bonus.

♦ **Panchakarma** refers to a particular prescription of cleansing the body from toxins through several procedures. Although this ancient practice once involved such invasive activities as enemas and forced vomiting, the modernized version is much more appealing. It involves detoxifying practices like steam baths, herbal oil massages, and a specialized diet. The purpose of these procedures is to let go of the toxins and to enhance your natural healing by preparing the body tissues to receive the benefits of nutrition and exercise. This can be an ideal ritual when you are experiencing an accumulation of *ama*, which is unmetabolized accumulated waste that is not used by the body. How would you know if you have accumulated *ama*? Check your tongue scraper: you might see a thick coating on your tongue. Alternately, you may experience body aches and pains, fatigue, and even a foggy mind. After you experience a panchakarma in a professional setting, you may be able to see ways to incorporate some of the rituals into your weekly routines.

Replace Products

Like my patient Bree, sometimes the first step is simply replacing certain toxic products with healthier ones. Here are a few of my favorite personal products:[20]

- *Dr. Bronner's* makes soap, cleaning products, detergent, and a number of other products made with organic and fair trade ingredients.

- *Beauty Counter* emphasizes its commitment to "clean" beauty and has created a "Never List" of over 1,800 ingredients commonly found in other beauty products which they commit not to use.

- *Eminence* produces face and body products using the power of plants; they grow most of the ingredients on their own certified, organic, sustainable farm, which has been researched for its beneficial properties.

- *Schmidt's* deodorant products are vegan, cruelty-free, and made with shea butter, coconut oil, and essential oils.

- *Vegamour* is a vegan shampoo and conditioner brand that strives to "optimize your hair's ecosystem," nourishing both the scalp and your hair follicles.

- *Saje* essential oils are a quality brand that I often use; "peppermint halo" is my go-to remedy for headaches. They have combined the active ingredient menthol, which has been shown to relieve pain topically and treat headaches and migraines.[21]

♦ Make your own! You can make a household cleanser using lemon and orange peels with vinegar. Many foods can be used as beauty products, like an oatmeal and avocado face mask. There are even recipes to make your own Ayurvedic sunscreen.

#CellCare: The benefits of a hair oil massage go far beyond nourishing your scalp. Hair oiling is a ritual rooted in science, originating from the Sanskrit word *sneha* which means to oil and love. The head is home to our senses and nervous system. In Ayurvedic practice, head massage is part of the daily routine to restore mental and physical balance. Among the recipes passed down in my family is hair growth oil. Try it out and let me know what you think.

Ingredients:

♦ 8 ounces organic coconut oil

♦ 10–12 fresh curry leaves, washed and dried

♦ 1 tablespoon black cumin seeds

♦ 2 tablespoons fenugreek seed

♦ 5 drops rosemary essential oil

To prepare hair oil:

- Grind black cumin seeds and fenugreek seeds into a fine powder.

- Heat coconut oil on low-medium flame.

- Add curry leaves and powder mixture into the coconut oil.

- Cook for 20 minutes, stirring every 2–3 minutes.

- Remove from heat and let it cool. Strain with cheesecloth.

- Store in an airtight glass bottle in a cool, dry spot. When the weather is cooler, it is natural for the oil to solidify.

- Apply to the scalp using your fingertips in a circular massaging motion. Use 2–3 times a week and keep in the hair at least 30 minutes before showering.

Incorporate Houseplants

Sometimes, places meant to be sources of comfort can build up toxins affecting our wellbeing. Surprisingly, most modern furnishings (like your sofa and mattress), synthetic materials (in your rugs and flooring), and stagnant air emit more chemicals than you might expect. Since these items are typically in enclosed spaces, these everyday pieces can increase indoor air pollution.

But here's the good news! NASA conducted a study back in 1989 that discovered that plants could absorb these harmful toxins from the air.[22] I highly recommend eating plants for the nutritional benefits, but there are many other ways we can benefit from household plants as well. Consider having two to three plants in eight-to-ten-inch pots for every 100 square feet. Not only will the plants help clean the air, but they can also increase our immune function,[23] concentration, productivity,[24] mood and reduce stress. Of course, all plants can purify the air to a certain degree, but here are some of the hardier ones that are easy to grow, even if you don't have a green thumb: aloe, monstera, pothos, money plant, snake plant, rosemary, and tulsi. All of these options are aesthetically pleasing, have multiple benefits, and will work to clean the air around you.

> **#CellCare:** *Tulsi* is one of my top choices because, not only can it help clarify the air, but you can eat it too! My mom is always trying to feed us tulsi, a.k.a. "holy basil." It's an adaptogen, meaning it can help the body adapt to stress, has anti-inflammatory properties, and can address the psychological, physiological, immunological, and metabolic stress of modern living.[25]

Eat More Fiber

Make sure your diet contains plenty of fiber to help your digestive system to remove toxins. Besides promoting healthy and regular bowel movements, high-fiber foods also bind with bile in the intestine, eliminating cholesterol, fat, and harmful toxins. As a result, toxins latch onto the fiber and are efficiently removed from your system. Refer to Chapter Four to be reminded of some great sources of fiber.

Drink More (Warm) Water

Hydration is one of the easiest (yet most overlooked) ways to remove toxins from your body and keep your detox organs (like the kidneys and the liver) happy. It's essential to focus on rehydrating first thing in the morning, after your body's been asleep for hours and hasn't had any new hydration. Drinking that first cup of water in the morning can help flush out toxins. Since you're not typically sweating or going to the bathroom while you sleep, your body doesn't have a chance to flush the toxins you're breathing in until you wake up and start to hydrate again. Warm water, in particular, stimulates peristalsis (movement in your GI tract), which in turn speeds up your metabolism, ultimately helping break down food and enhance absorption of nutrients. One study found that switching from cold water to warm water can even help with weight loss.[26] Water also helps flush excess caffeine, sugar, and toxin. The amount of water your body needs to remove toxins every day will vary from person to person. Use your body as a guide. Pay attention to how your digestion is working, how your skin and muscles feel, and how your mind is functioning.

Find ways to layer drinking water on preexisting habits throughout the day. For example, if you typically have a coffee or tea in the morning, try to drink a glass of water before your caffeinated beverage. (Your body naturally produces cortisol in the morning, which helps you wake up, but caffeine blunts the effectiveness of that hormone, possibly because of its effect on your body's vitamins and minerals.)

Sometimes water can just be plain boring, so I will often add lemons, limes, mint leaves, crushed ginger, cucumbers, or pineapple. I turn these into flavored ice cubes and add them to my water. I recommend drinking water at room temperature (once the ice cube has melted and flavored the water). Ayurveda recommends room-temperature water for digestion; it keeps your digestive fire—*agni*—active. You can think of agni is the force of intelligence that drives every cell, every tissue, and every system within your body. Cold water "puts out" that digestive fire.

> **#CellCare:** One of the most game-changing teas I use is from a blend of culinary spices. Using a combination of cumin, coriander, and fennel, the tea relieves gastric bloating and indigestion; it also helps stimulate *agni*, helps your body absorb nutrients, and soothes inflammation in the stomach lining. Each of these spices comes with its own

benefits. Cumin can help flush out toxic waste, ultimately improving elimination. Coriander can improve digestion, absorption, and calm muscle spasms accompanying gastric discomfort. Lastly, fennel supports moving our lymphatics and relaxing the digestive tract. You can enjoy this tea multiple times throughout the day.

To prepare the "CCF" tea blend:

♦   6 Tablespoons cumin seeds

♦   6 Tablespoons coriander seeds

♦   6 Tablespoons fennel seeds

♦   Mix and store in an airtight glass jar.

To prepare one cup of tea:

♦   Boil 1 ¼ cup of water and add one teaspoon of CCF blend.

♦   Boil the tea for 5 to 10 minutes. Strain the seeds and enjoy.

Remove Pesticides from Your Produce

The best way to reduce your exposure to pesticides is to buy USDA Organic, which is grown without the use of synthetic pesticides. Alternately, if you can't find fresh organic produce or don't want to suffer the extra cost, you can check out your freezer section. Look for frozen organic produce, which is cost effective, frozen at its peak ripeness, and easy to incorporate into meals.

If you buy nonorganic produce and want to do your best to wash off the residual pesticides, here are three easy and cheap ways to clean your produce at home. (In fact, I use the saltwater soak on my organic produce as well to clean off any leftover residue. They're quick and easy!)

- **Saltwater soak:** Research suggests that soaking fruits and vegetables in a 10 percent saltwater solution for twenty minutes gets rid of most of the residues from the four most common pesticides.[27] This is the one I usually do as I am washing my greens before draining them in my salad spinner.

- **Vinegar soak:** Vinegar is another way to remove residues from fruits and vegetables. You can make a solution of four-parts water to one-part vinegar and soak for about twenty minutes. Vinegar can also remove many types of bacteria that may be found on food as well.

- **Baking soda soak:** Recent research shows us an additional option, which may include submerging your produce in one teaspoon of baking soda with two cups of water for at least five minutes.[28] The longer you soak, the more chemicals will come off. Then, rinse again in tap water before eating.

Unfortunately, using store-bought vegetable cleaners has been shown to be no more effective than soaking in regular water. So, save your money for where it counts.

You may also consider trying to grow your own. I have become a hydroponic farmer (which means I don't need to get my hands dirty) and grow all my greens in a tower and my microgreens right on my kitchen counter.

Bathing Rituals

Taking a shower or a hot bath is always good self-care, but you can add on these two bathing rituals to help your body detoxify. Remember to avoid products that are scented with anything other than essential oils:

◆ **Epsom salt baths** will help draw out toxins through your skin, ease muscle soreness, and as a bonus, often help improve sleep. My favorite reason for adding at least one Epsom salt bath to my weekly ritual is the extra magnesium I receive, which helps manage physical and mental stress.[29] Here is my go-to evening bath recipe:

◇ 2 cups Epsom salts

◇ 10 drops bergamot essential oil

◇ ½ cup organic unrefined olive oil

♦ **Hydrotherapy** works by alternating hot and cold water in the shower. For example, after two minutes of warm water, turn the shower to cold for thirty seconds. The alternating temperatures help decrease inflammation and stimulate your blood flow. Remember, one of your body's chief pathways of toxin removal is through the blood, so your stimulated circulation will help remove those toxins from your body. If you're courageous, you can get these same benefits from cold-water swimming or ice baths. I once enjoyed an invigorating hydrotherapy experience at Bota-Bota, a floating boat spa in Montreal, which guides guests through different baths of varying temperatures, creating an entire water circuit. If you ever happen to be in Montreal, it's an inexpensive way to treat yourself! However, you can create your own hydrotherapy circuits at home. The experience of moving through hot and cold water ultimately repairs and soothes your mind and body.

Sweating Rituals

Yes, I am recommending you try to get hot and sweaty regularly. By sweating, your body purges all kinds of toxins, including heavy metals, especially from fatty tissues.

♦ **Exercise.** Help your skin purge toxins by making sweaty exercise a regular part of your life. Exercise also helps increase your circulation and blood flow, another toxin-removal win. If you want to work up a sweat, try hot yoga. The heat will help you limber up while enabling you to purge toxins simultaneously. But even if you're not ready to enter the yoga studio, you can turn on your favorite music and break a good sweat dancing like no one is watching.

◆ **Saunas**—especially infrared saunas—are another option to help you sweat it out. Research found that "sauna bathing is associated with a reduction in the risk of vascular diseases, such as high blood pressure and cardiovascular disease, neurocognitive diseases, nonvascular conditions, such as pulmonary diseases, mental health disorders, and mortality. Furthermore, sauna bathing alleviated skin diseases, arthritis, headache, and flu conditions. The evidence also suggests that regular sauna baths are associated with a better health-related quality of life."[30] Consider using the sauna at your gym or invest in an in-home sauna.

Healthy Living App

The Environmental Working Group, as highlighted before, created an app called "EWG's Healthy Living" that provides the EWG's ratings for food, personal care, and cleaning products. It's a great tool that enables you to scan products at the store while you shop, helping you easily identify the level of toxicity in most common products. The app will assign a simple grade to a product—high hazard, medium hazard, or low hazard—and allows you to further examine what ingredients are harmful. This can help you get familiar with some of the most common offenders in your most-used products—such as phthalates, parabens, and triclosan—and enable you to fill your grocery cart with products you can feel good about.

Massage for Toxin Removal

When we feel pain or soreness in our muscles, it may signify lactic acid build up; this is a naturally occurring compound our body produces, but when it builds up, it can cause pain. We sometimes get accumulated lactic acid after a hard workout; your body knows how to flush this naturally, but a massage can help. Massage can break down this compound and remove it from the body by increasing blood and lymph circulation. In addition, the relaxation of the soft tissue (muscle, connective tissue, tendons, ligaments) releases tension and helps reduce the adverse effects of stress. Plus, it feels great!

WORTH THE EFFORT

Sometimes when I get to this point with my patients, they heave a deep sigh. It seems like a lot of work: I know. Toxins are seemingly omnipresent, and it can feel almost futile to try to avoid them.

However, it gets easier with each step. I love seeing my patients start by making small lifestyle adjustments that lead to consistent changes in their body's intake of toxins. A decision to replace plastic Tupperware with glass, for instance, or opting for a new beauty product with only clean ingredients instead of buying the same old toxic brand—these are momentary decisions. Still, they have a long-term effect on what your body takes in.

It may seem like a steep hill to climb at first—to read all the ingredient labels, to enter each product into Environmental Working Group's website—but over time, you'll learn what brands you like. *After that, it gets easier*—I promise.

Sometimes my patients ask me how consistent I am with following these rules. They want to know if I *never* consume high-fructose corn syrup, use plastic, or go on walks near any location that uses pesticides. I admit—I don't avoid toxins perfectly; I don't think anyone does. For instance, my neighborhood walks take me past some pesticide-treated lawns—but they also get me sunshine, exercise, and a mental boost from being out in nature. When I'm in the mood to get ice cream, I'll get a pint of dairy-free chocolate peanut butter—but I read the label first to make sure it's made of natural ingredients, or even make it at home!

Why is it worth the effort to read ingredient labels, change some lifestyle habits, and swap out some products for others? Because when you remove toxic elements in your environment, you can improve your cellular health, which is the foundation for health, beauty, and longevity.

Reflect on Your #CellCare

Using these guiding questions, take a moment to build self-awareness and reflect on the presence of toxins in your life:

♦ Are you sensitive to personal care products, like body wash, lotions, shampoos, conditioners, cosmetics, or shaving cream?

♦ Do you often eat nonorganic food (including animal products) that contain GMOs, processed ingredients, and additives?

♦ Do you drink sodas, juices, or other beverages with natural or refined sweeteners or artificial sweeteners?

♦ Do you use standard cleaning products and scented products? Do you use chemical-heavy products like paints, glues, varnishes, herbicides, or pesticides? Do you regularly visit areas that may have been treated with pesticides or chemicals, such as golf courses or farms?

♦ Does your home have signs of mold or water damage? Are you exposed to air pollutants like pesticides from nearby agricultural farms, industrial pollution from freeways, or fumes from gas or propane stoves?

♦ Reference the shaded box titled "Do You Have a Toxicity Problem?" Are you aware that these symptoms might be linked to a toxin burden in your body?

DESIGN YOUR WELLBEING

If you answered yes to one or more of the above questions, this area might be one you want to target for improvement by incorporating some detoxifying rituals. In the space below, note your thoughts about your toxicity exposure. Then, name a ritual you may want to incorporate into your life.

8

SPACE AS SANCTUARY

"Outer order contributes to inner calm."

~ GRETCHEN RUBIN, AUTHOR

JOANNA WAS THE BREADWINNER IN HER FAMILY; SHE CARED for her two teenage kids and ran her entire household. Her husband traveled for work and was often gone for extended periods. As a result, she was constantly running from here to there—going to work, driving her kids to activities, trying to squeeze in errands. She told me, "Life is so hectic. I constantly feel on edge; I'm run down, anxious, and always depleted. I just have way too much on my plate."

While she was sharing this on a video call, I couldn't help noticing the room behind her. Piles were stacked on her counters and there was a heap of laundry on the floor. Gently, I asked her, "Do you feel like your physical space is helping or exacerbating your stress?"

Her living space was—in her words—"total chaos." There was not a hint of organization in her home, and items were rarely put away in their proper place. When her family ran out of essentials like milk, no one seemed to know. The counters were covered with mail and unopened Amazon packages; her kitchen table was cluttered with magazines, books, and school projects. There wasn't even a place for the family to sit down and have a meal together. Joanna often mentioned the chaotic atmosphere of her house to me when she explained her reasons for feeling stressed.

Joanna had recently accepted a new position that required her to go back and forth between her home and downtown. Although it was a great job, her commute threw a new wrench into the gears. As Joanna explained, she wasn't organized enough to pack lunch or snacks. Instead, she would come home and eat whatever she could heat in the microwave because she didn't plan her meals. This lack of planning and organization also affected her kids; they did the same thing, eating whatever was quickly available, which often meant a frozen pizza. Joanna also told me that she was not sleeping well. I wondered if her bedroom was similar to what she'd said to me about her kitchen: cluttered and unorganized.

We began our work by assessing the different aspects of her wellbeing. For example, I often see that nutrition's impact on health with my patients is often misunderstood and underestimated. So, we started by making sure Joanna had easily accessible, healthy foods to take to work. Then, we talked about getting her living space organized, not only for herself but also for the wellbeing of her family.

At first, she was hesitant to make changes because it seemed too complicated. But about halfway in, Joanna finally told me she was ready to get to work. She could no longer go on living the way she was. Her disorganized space was impacting her health more than she had realized. After she began organizing her living space, she felt more energized and told me, "The changes make me feel amazing." She felt a sense of calm when she didn't waste twenty minutes looking for her keys in the morning. She had more energy because she was fueling her body with the food it needed and also sleeping better as she created a new bedtime ritual.

PHYSICAL SPACE MATTERS

Let's say you are invited over to a friend's house to taste her latest matcha latte recipe. You walk in and are suddenly stumbling over packages at the door and trash waiting to be thrown out, with nowhere to put your purse and coat. After a few moments, you make your way to the kitchen, only to be greeted by a sink full of dishes and an island full of mail. As you clean off a place to sit, your sense of calm and excitement about this afternoon is overtaken by the chaos that surrounds you.

Alternatively, imagine heading over to this same friend's house and feeling like you're on a mini staycation upon entering. You're greeted with a fresh, inviting, and clean entryway, with a spot to hang your coat and purse. There's no stumbling here—just simply entering the kitchen where your friend is excited to show you what she's creating. You pull up a seat at the island as she presents to you her matcha tastings. The room smells of lavender wafting from the diffuser in the corner, and your tea is served in a clean mug and tastes delicious. You feel calm and excited to spend your afternoon and are ready to catch up on life.

If we're being honest, most of us would admit to feeling unease in a messy, cluttered space. There is a reason we love going to spas and hotels to be pampered, yet somehow, we overlook the value of creating this kind of space for ourselves.

Clutter and mess can be cumulative. For example, your bedroom closet may be so full you can't find anything, yet you continue to stuff clothes in the closet. Maybe you have mail piled up so high that you don't remember the last bill you paid or don't know when the next batch is due. You might have a messy kitchen drawer with anything and everything in it—so what happens when you need to find something?

Creating and maintaining a clean, organized physical space doesn't mean your home will always be clean. Messes will always pop up—but you can use rituals to help keep them under control. For example, I dislike doing dishes, and sometimes they pile up in my sink. But I have a ritual so the pile doesn't get out of hand: if I'm waiting for water to boil or something is cooking on the stove, I'll clean the dishes in the sink while I'm waiting. I also dislike folding laundry, but I get around that by dumping out the washed laundry on my bed as I'm prepping for my evening bath ritual. While the bathtub is filling, I will fold away, knowing that in less than ten minutes I'm going to be relaxing in an Epsom salt bath. (For more ideas about how to make housework more enjoyable, look ahead to the "Mindful Housework" ritual.)

Clutter = Cortisol

Imagine this scenario. You live in a cluttered home, and suddenly the electricity goes out. You need a flashlight. You know you have one, but you don't know where it is. Everyone in your household starts to search through the mess in the dark. You're yelling at each other, barking orders, and trying to hear one another from across the house. Finally, someone finds the flashlight. It becomes apparent as soon as you turned on the button that the batteries are dead. Now, you have to search for batteries. The collective searching, yelling, complaining, and fumbling around in the dark resumes.

By the time you manage to come up with a working flashlight, you and your family might have wasted an hour. Whenever you can't find something, the frustration of that moment shifts your body into a low-grade fight or flight mode, which bathes your system in cortisol, the stress hormone. Studies have shown that when people perceive their homes as cluttered, they have a depressed mood over the course of a day.[1]

Remember—cortisol is not necessarily the bad guy. As you now know, cortisol is the hormone that helps you become alert when you wake up. Furthermore, cortisol regulates blood sugar levels, blood pressure, and helps maintain proper brain-body communication. When released at the appropriate times and in the right amounts, cortisol can be beneficial.

But when you experience *chronic* low-grade stress—which a disorganized space can perpetuate—the constant cortisol can cause wear and tear on the body. A continuous release of cortisol causes inflammation, weakening your immune system and leading to all kinds of symptoms, including headaches, joint pain, hormonal imbalances, and weight gain. In addition, chronic low-grade stress makes you more prone to infections and even autoimmune diseases.

Trust me on this: your brain likes organization. The brain appreciates rituals; it doesn't want to think any more than it already has to. On the other hand, clutter drains the brain because clutter is a distraction—it reduces your ability to be productive and your working memory.

You're more likely to get a task done in less time when you have a clear plan. Conversely, completing a task can be more time-consuming and stressful when you don't have a plan. The same concept applies to your living and working space: if your space is disorganized, finding things will be more time-consuming, and you'll experience unnecessary stress. For example, consider how often you have lost the remote control between the sofa cushions. However, an organized, decluttered space can improve your focus, lower your stress, and help you experience greater overall wellbeing.

Experiencing frustration because of clutter may not seem like a big deal, but all those moments of cortisol-releasing stress can take a toll over time. A disorganized or stress-inducing living space can negatively impact your mind and body, leaving you anxious or depressed.[2] Whether at work or home, a cluttered environment can make you feel overwhelmed. Walking into a messy kitchen may not inspire you to cook for yourself and you may be less likely to exercise if your Peloton has turned into a drying rack. As Joanna found in her own life, these disorganized spaces can affect the wellbeing of your entire family. But by the same token, your physical environment is an area where small improvements can make a big impact for those sharing your living space.

Why Get Organized?

If all of that doesn't get your attention, consider some of the benefits of organizing your space:

◆ **Getting organized can save you time** because it will be easier to find things when you have a place to put them away. Plus, when there's a power outage, you'll know exactly where to find the flashlight and batteries!

◆ **Getting organized can save you money**. Think of the dollars you can save when you don't have to buy something you already have because you can't find it. For instance, you know you had an iPhone charger somewhere but have now misplaced it. So of course, the easiest thing to do is buy another one, let the other one collect dust in a corner somewhere, and create demand for unnecessary production. Unfortunately, not only does that waste your money, but it creates environmental waste as well.

◆ **Getting organized makes you calmer and less stressed**. Less cortisol means your body can more frequently enjoy the calm of your parasympathetic state. You'll also be able to focus on the activities and people you want to focus on, rather than being distracted by the stress of a chaotic environment.

◆ **Getting organized can help you be more fit**.[3] People who have cleaner homes tend to exercise more, although researchers are still looking to pinpoint why that might be. Most of us might have an anecdotal idea: when you're living in a cluttered space, it can be easy to feel overwhelmed; rather than physically moving your body, you're more inclined to lay low. (Remember that Peloton covered with drying clothes—it's a very expensive drying rack!) But when you're in a clean, organized space, your mind is free to do other nice things for yourself—such as getting outside for a workout. Researchers also speculated that cleaning up can be a good work out in and of itself!

♦ **Getting organized decreases procrastination and increases productivity.**[4] When you work at a messy desk, sometimes it's hard to be productive and efficient. You don't know where to start, so you procrastinate. If you are a master procrastinator, you may not realize that your disorganized state may also affect your decisiveness and your overall satisfaction with life. But when you come into a clean space, you're ready to get the work done!

♦ **Getting organized can help you focus.** If you have trouble getting your to-do list accomplished or finishing a project, spending a few minutes organizing your things can make it easier to get your work done. Studies even demonstrate that people can process information better in an uncluttered and organized workspace and be more productive, less distracted, and less irritable.[5]

Here's another way to think about it: the space we create for ourselves is often a reflection of our personality and an indication of self-respect. This is one reason why potential employers usually expect job applicants to look well-groomed and professionally dressed: our external appearance can indicate inner preparedness and confidence. The same may be true for our personal spaces. A cluttered, chaotic, or disorganized space could suggest that your health and happiness are not a priority. However, although other tasks may feel more important, your physical space will influence your ability to effectively function in all other areas of your life. Even if you don't believe that for yourself, you might still be aware of how others could negatively perceive you if they see a chaotic home environment.

Messy spaces can have some detrimental effects on your interpersonal relationships. If you live in a household where your spouse is always leaving their dirty socks around, that can trigger unnecessary stress and tension in the relationship. Over time, the daily habits that may not bother the person doing them can create stress for the other people they live with. In addition, the cluttered spaces impact our emotional state, which we will see in the next chapter is a critical component to holistic wellbeing.

In other ways, our physical space has an impact on our lifespan. People tend to have a healthier diet when they live in a clean and organized environment.[6] When you open your refrigerator and you can clearly see fruits and vegetables as opposed to a jumble of takeout containers and half-used condiment jars, you may be more inclined to eat fresh food rather than days-old leftovers. In this way, your space can reflect your inner state, but it can also *motivate* your internal state. Clean spaces also help your health because they reduce allergens, which—as we discussed in Chapter Seven—can add to a toxic burden.

Ultimately, external calm can aid your relational health, lead to greater physical wellbeing, and promote inner peace. That's why the opposite of a chaotic environment is a healing space.

Healing Spaces

Healing Spaces is a term coined by the Samueli Institute, a center for Integrative Medicine. These spaces evoke a sense of cohesion of the mind, body, and spirit. Specifically, an Optimal Healing Environment (OHE) is a space where healing occurs by addressing all aspects of a person's individuality. A healing space intentionally considers the physical, social, psychological, and spiritual characteristics of the people who will reside in that space and creates design elements that will enhance their distinctive wellbeing.

For example, let's consider what a healing home space might look like for a yoga teacher who wants to optimize her small New York City apartment. Her physical space, is filled with smaller, multi-functional furniture pieces that don't overpower the 300 square feet she lives in, like a fold dining table that can double as a desk. Her social space consists of plush floor cushions and a day bed; the cushions can be stacked when she wants more room for yoga. In her psychologic space, she uses sheer window coverings to maximize natural light; she places indoor plants on the window sills to improve the air quality and add color; and she diffuses essential oils to create pleasing aromas. Lastly, the nook where she retreats to nurture her spiritual side is equipped with a comfy armchair and a floor lamp.

Anyone can create a healing space, even if you don't feel particularly creative. Whether you're dealing with a 300–square foot apartment or a 3,000–square foot house, you can design an oasis that you are happy to return to each day by considering what will best enhance these areas: physical space, social considerations, and your psychological and spiritual wellbeing.

In her famous book, *Spark Joy*, Marie Kondo recommends that a healing space be decluttered and free of objects that don't make you feel happy.[7] This may require you to move magazines, papers, and anything that doesn't evoke peace or calm feelings. Try starting out by creating a healing space in a single room; later, you might feel ready to apply these concepts to your entire home. Consider your home your personal sanctuary.

> **#CellCare:** Here's a straightforward process you can use to declutter a stress-inducing space. When cleaning out an area, ask yourself if you want to keep something, give it away, sell it, or throw it out. To help yourself answer that question, consider: "Is this something I need, something I love, or something I actually use?" If the answer is no, move it out.

SPACE VILLAINS

Besides clutter, there are certain negative environmental elements that can consistently make a space more stressful to be in. I'm a huge science fiction fan, so I'm going to call these space villains.

- **Fluorescent lighting:** Fluorescent bulbs can have a harmful UV range that strain the eyes; in fact, fluorescent lighting can increase UV-related eye diseases such as cataracts.[8] These lights work through a very rapid flicker, which may not be visually apparent, but our brain can still perceive it, setting off neurological stress. Some of the indirect effects caused by fluorescent lights include migraines, eyestrain, sleep issues, stress, and, anxiety. It's also fairly obvious that fluorescent lighting is unappealing! It's more likely to remind you of a stressful workplace than a healing sanctuary.

- **Dust:** It's never good for us to inhale dust; it's an environmental toxin and will negatively impact your health. You should open your windows to let air circulate throughout your home. As discussed in the previous chapter, allergens from furniture dust can also be bad. Vacuuming and dusting frequently can help keep your space dust-free.

- **Paint and toxic furniture:** Certain types of paint can be toxic, so be careful when selecting paint colors for your home. Many baby furniture manufacturers now have their products green-certified to give parents reassurance that their furniture is nontoxic. Also, consider what colors you choose to integrate and make sure they align deliberately for each space. Colors can easily become space villains if they're not used intentionally. Dark colors can help simulate nighttime, which might make them appropriate for the bedroom, but they may not suit your home office.

♦ **Disorganized piles:** It can be easy to let mail pile up on the counter or laundry to pile up in the corner of the living room. Sometimes this is okay, but over time, these piles can keep growing, eventually overtaking an entire area and making it hard to do anything productive there. You can try to keep these piles at a minimum by doing one of the rituals like the "20 Minute Pick-Up."

SPACE HEROES

No good science fiction movie is complete without heroes to fight back the villains. Fortunately, there are more space heroes than villains, and they can restore order to your personal universe.

Light

Natural light is beautiful, and it also helps regulate your circadian rhythm. As we discussed in Chapter Six, although the circadian rhythm is most often associated with sleep, it's responsible for regulating a wide range of your body's processes. Exposing yourself to natural light can help you align with that rhythm. So as much as possible, orient your main living time near windows and pull back those curtains.

If you can't have natural light in your space, soft lighting is recommended. Ayurvedic practitioners recommend using soft (not fluorescent) lighting and full-spectrum lights in the winter when there's less sunlight to counteract seasonal affective disorder and depression.[9] Seasonal affective disorder is a mood disorder that can be triggered by insufficient light; although the cause is unknown, it appears to be linked to your circadian rhythm. Alternatively, consider light box therapy, which can mimic outdoor light. It is thought that this specific type of light can ease symptoms of this disorder and lift your mood due to a chemical shift in your brain.

> **#CellCare:** If you live in a part of the world that frequently gets long, dark days, or if you're in an environment that doesn't allow you exposure to much natural light, a light box will make for a good investment. The light box should provide 10,000 lux of light exposure to mimic the sun's rays. It is best to use it in the morning for about twenty to thirty minutes to help align your circadian rhythm.

Chromotherapy

Chromotherapy is a practice based around the idea that colors produce various electrical impulses in your brain and these impulses stimulate hormonal and biochemical processes.[10] As we've previously discussed, your hormones and chemistry can impact your entire body. Some colors are more stimulating, whereas others cue your body to relax.

This is not a widely accepted theory in Western medicine. However, we've all experienced the effects that colors have on us and can recognize that certain colors evoke different feelings.

Here are some common effects of different colors:

COLOR THERAPY

RED
Brings energy to all organs and stimulates passion and spontaneity

VIOLET
Stimulates artistic qualities, self-knowlege, intuition, and meditation

ORANGE
Linked with optimism, creativity, and productivity

WHITE
Brings spiritual healing, protection, and inspiration

BLUE
Calming, stimulates parasympathetic nervous system

YELLOW
Stimulates joy, happiness, and emotional well-being

GREEN
Linked to nature, regulates the pituitary gland, and relieves stress

When you're thinking about what colors you might want to employ in your spaces, consider the colors that you enjoy most out in nature. It's no surprise that colors like black and dark brown tend to elicit feelings of sadness; we associate those colors with failing plants and death. However, colors like green make us think of flourishing nature and health; blue and violet are calming colors for the parasympathetic system and great for meditation; and yellow and orange can stimulate creativity and joy.

Consider incorporating colors as accents to create a home that feels like an oasis without being overstimulating. By becoming aware of your surroundings, you can intentionally maintain a sense of calm.

Scent

Scent can be very powerful. When we breathe in, our sense of smell is activated and the surrounding floating molecules enter our nose. They rush through our nostrils and attach to the olfactory cilia, which transports the smell into the olfactory bulb above and behind the nose at the base of our brain. These bulbs, which look like small lima bean structures, encompass cells that interpret, amplify, and transmit a chemical message to the limbic system.[11]

Since the limbic system is the seat of memory and emotion, it translates memories from scents into real sensations and impressions. As a result, the smell of funnel cake conjures up childhood memories of going to the fair, or the smell of suntan lotion reminds you of your beach holiday. Our sense of smell is connected to our memories and emotions.

Hospitals usually smell sterile, with scents of alcohol or bleach cleaners. However, some hospitals today are transforming their environments into healing spaces. Many facilities infuse pleasant aromas like the ocean air and freshly baked cookies to create a calming and healing environment since sterile smells don't create a relaxing environment.

Consider which smells help you feel calm, happy, and relaxed. Perhaps it's the smell of pine, like the woods where you grew up; maybe it's a smell of something delicious baking in the oven. Look for ways to incorporate natural scents, like essential oils, flowers, spices, or cooking. By incorporating these familiar and calming scents into your space, you can help lower your stress and maintain a greater sense of calm and wellbeing.

#**CellCare:** Proceed with caution when it comes to scented candles. Many candles are made from paraffin wax, which is a byproduct of petroleum; when you burn the candle, it's releasing harmful chemicals into the air. Additionally, burning scented candles can release compounds like formaldehyde, which is a known carcinogen. However, there are many natural candle options made with soy or coconut wax and essential oils that can be a great addition to your home.

Nature

Including nature in your space is another way to create a relaxing environment. You can do this by hanging pictures of nature, putting potted plants in your space, or simply letting natural light into your home or office. When the weather allows, try opening a window and taking in the view and the sounds from outside.

Having plants in your everyday space is deeply healing because plants are living things. In Chapter Seven, we discussed the ways plants can help clean the air in a space by absorbing toxins. However, they also have a powerful positive effect on your mood and physical health. Your immune system, mood, and productivity are enhanced, and your stress levels are reduced. One of my favorite elements in my own space is a hanging herb garden. It looks different every day, and it's incredibly soothing to look at. Every time I walk by, it's like seeing life in motion.

Many studies attest to the varied benefits of plants. For example, a study in the *Journal of Physiologic Anthropology* showed that plants can reduce stress levels and make you feel more comfortable.[12] Another study did brain scans of students who studied with real, live plants in the classroom, and it showed they were more attentive and better able to concentrate than students in other groups.[13]

Other research found that the presence of flowers, green plants, and other natural materials positively impacted the autonomic nervous system, leading to an increased parasympathetic response—a.k.a. relaxation.[14] Still another study showed that plants in the workplace increased productivity and reduced the number of employees' sick days.[15] It's time to go get yourself a plant or two! Artificial plants can also improve mood and morale for those without green thumbs.

Organization

Last but not least, let's come back to organization, our strongest defense against the space villain of clutter.

To stay organized, I recommend going minimal. To set up your workspace, you'll need a computer, keyboard, pen, notebook, and possibly a desk calendar. Use the wall space for pictures of loved ones or pleasing nature scenes. You don't need much more than that. Do your best to keep your desk clear of random papers. As much as possible, either file, recycle, or process those papers to keep your workspace clear.

Use the few items in your workspace to help you stay organized. For example, I have a yearly planner with monthly and weekly sections on my desk where I can write my priority tasks. I write the top three tasks for each day, and when I'm done, I check them off. (I've already admitted that I love to check off boxes after accomplishing a task!)

Writing down and keeping track of my tasks for the week gives me a sense of calm, and crossing off completed tasks is a way for me to affirm my day's efforts. It also helps me gauge if I need to make changes in the way I plan my schedule. Did I check off all the boxes? Did I overbook or under-book myself? Did I do too much, or could I do a little bit more? The simple task of checking off those tasks helps me evaluate my productivity and workload.

This method of task organization can also help you determine how your schedule makes you feel. For instance, if you're a person who has trouble saying no and you're feeling run down, a written list of your weekly tasks can help you identify which activities were too much. In addition, that record can help you figure out which specific tasks or commitments you need to say no to in the future.

When we're struggling or going through a difficult time, we're quick to forget our accomplishments, but looking back at your calendar will help you see that you were productive. Of course, it's human nature for us to just remember the negative, but a calendar on your desk can create a positive tracking system. This will allow you opportunities to affirm your hard work. So go ahead: pat yourself on the back!

THE CHALLENGES OF CREATING A HEALING SPACE

There are plenty of potential objections to putting in the effort to declutter your living space—so let's address them.

"I'm just a messy person."

Some people may believe they are just messy by nature. Or because they are creative and artistic, they think they need a cluttered space to thrive. If you fall into this category, I invite you to deeply consider the following questions:

◆ Does your creativity truly flow best in a messy environment? Is it possible for your creativity to thrive in a more peaceful and organized environment?

◆ Are you sleeping well at night? Are you tired? Is it possible your chaotic living environment prevents you from getting quality sleep?

- How are your relationships? Do you feel free to invite people into your space? Do you avoid hosting people at your house because you're embarrassed about the mess?

Sometimes, a contained mess may not affect other areas of a person's life. For instance, an art studio might be a messy space, but if the rest of the artist's house is clean and organized, that one messy area likely won't be a concern.

Consider the various factors of your lifestyle and health to determine if messy areas might be affecting you. Do you need to wash a dish every time you sit to eat? Is your kitchen table a place to dine or a place to set things? Can you easily navigate your closet? Do you often find yourself searching for items you regularly use, like your keys or cell phone? If your stress is regularly provoked and your wellbeing is compromised due to the disorganization in your living space, then the excuse that you're just a messy person isn't serving you. Remember the power of your neuroplasticity: reshape your mind and transform your life.

"My roommate/spouse/partner is a messy person."

Maybe the mess that's driving you crazy isn't your own at all—it's generated by your much beloved living companion. Often, the people you live with may not even realize their untidiness is negatively affecting you both. Try addressing this challenge by having an honest conversation about how the lack of organization impacts your mood—feel free to share some of the research in this chapter about the physical effects of living in a stressful space.

Then, get practical. Try to identify the spaces that are most significant for your shared wellbeing and strategize ways to keep them clean. For instance, if you're sharing a bedroom, acknowledge that a decluttered space can help promote peaceful sleep and is an area to prioritize effort. Maybe "gamify" keeping the room organized by turning pick-up sessions into a competition, or assign each person certain responsibilities in keeping the room clean and come up with a fun reward system for success.

There's also great relief in finding ways to retreat to your own personal areas. If possible, assign each other private spaces that can be free of the others' (loving) influence.

"I have young kids."

Young children can be messy (in fact, plenty of big children can be messy!), and it may be challenging to keep your space clean if you have dynamic little ones making messes in your wake. If you are able, try setting up a designated space where they can play. That area can contain the mess, preventing it from taking over the rest of your living space. For example, you could try to contain the toys in a playpen or a child's room. If they have their own room, you can choose to close the door and not worry about what's behind it.

Recruit older children as partners in your mission against the mess. Enlist their help coming up with organizational systems. For example, make an event out of purging your closets together. Help them identify ways they can organize their different spaces. Consider developing a reward system that recognizes their efforts to keep the home picked up.

I realize not everyone has the luxury of designating a separate space for children, but there are ways to keep your space tidy, even when existing in small spaces with young children. For example, try taking out just one toy or book at a time for each child and have them do the same thing themselves. This also teaches them to focus on one task at a time, rather than being distracted by endless toy options or expecting that they can always have more.

If it's too much to expect your young children to participate in cleaning efforts, the adults in your home can spend five minutes putting things away after the kids go to sleep for the night. This can help prevent the mess from getting out of hand. Think of it as maintenance of the space.

"Minimalism is not my style."

What about personal preferences? While contemporary style centers around a clean, minimal aesthetic, some people prefer a lot of decorations; this can be especially true for older generations. Perhaps your preferred aesthetic is to have a home filled with knick-knacks and figurines, with walls and mantles covered in family photos, paintings, and other pictures. If those family pictures bring you comfort, then this aesthetic isn't one you need to change. On the contrary, the pictures and decorations might legitimately contribute to your wellbeing.

However, there is a fine line between having décor for comfort and hoarding. Hoarders may struggle with their mental or physical wellbeing or even feel slightly ashamed of the condition of their

THE ANATOMY OF WELLBEING

space, which can prevent them from engaging in healthy social relationships. If you have a lot of items in your living space and you're beginning to feel distracted or stressed by the clutter, it's time to purge. Consider enlisting a friend or loved one to help you through this process.

"Making changes to my space would be too expensive."

I'm giving a lot of advice about decorating and arranging space, but I know not everyone can afford the space they want. Perhaps your income requires you to live in a small apartment, or there's a bright neon sign right across the street shining into your window every evening. What can you do if your living space doesn't lend itself to being much of a sanctuary?

In these cases, when you create your space, focus on items that are meaningful to you. Pick objects that remind you of a vacation you enjoyed or photographs that have special memories attached to them. You don't necessarily have to buy new things. Just make sure you are comfortable in the space and that you can put things away after you take them out for use. And if you're able to put any plants in your space, I recommend you do so. You can often find plants and pots being given away on sites like Offer Up.

A cluttered space can lead to a stressful environment, impacting our health in ways we normally wouldn't consider. Thankfully, there are many small steps that can be taken to transform your space into a sanctuary.

308

RITUALS FOR
HEALING SPACES

Intentional practices around your environment can positively impact your wellbeing. Let's talk about some of the rituals that can help promote peace and tranquility.

Optimize Your Work Space

When setting up your workspace, position your desk so that it faces a window rather than a wall. In the case of an office or work space without any windows, display a picture of nature above or next to your desk instead. The addition of flowers and plants can enhance a space and purify the air. It is still possible to bring some nature into your work environment, even if you work in a basement or dark location. A lucky bamboo could be a good choice, for instance.

Clear the clutter from your workspace using some of the suggestions from earlier in this chapter so that it's clean and organized. When you don't have natural light in your space, try using phototherapy lights to simulate sunlight.

Organize to Minimize Chaos

An organized space makes your belongings easily accessible—both for you and everyone else who engages in your space. Here are a few ways I try to keep my spaces organized:

♦ My closet is organized according to color and season. By having an organized closet, it's easy for me to choose clothes, and friends who want to borrow clothes know exactly where to find them.

♦ I dedicate certain days to cleaning tasks. One day per month, I clean the entire house. One day per week, I do the laundry. By following this ritual, I avoid falling behind and experiencing stress from living in a messy home.

♦ My grains, beans, and dry goods are kept in glass jars so that I can find exactly what I'm looking for. For easy visibility of fruits and vegetables, I have clear organizers in my refrigerator. Having these helps me see when items are running low, so I know what I need to buy at the supermarket next time.

Embrace Mundane Housework

Maybe the thought of getting organized sounds unpleasant. After all, most of us are used to dreading chores. But research shows that if you do chores with some intention behind them, they can turn into a mood boost.

One study found that, "people who were mindful when washing dishes—in other words they took the time to smell the soap and to take in the experience—reported a 27 percent reduction in nervousness, along with a 25 percent improvement in 'mental inspiration.'"[16] Practicing mindfulness when doing housework like folding laundry or doing the dishes can actually help your body create presence and self-awareness.

310

Alternately, put on a great dance playlist while cleaning the bathroom, or listen to an interesting podcast or audio book while cleaning out your fridge. Try watching a show you like while folding laundry or ironing.

Chores are something we often put off because we don't enjoy them, but there are meaningful and fun rituals you can implement that can actually make the experience enjoyable. As a bonus—you'll be living in a cleaner, more organized space!

Aromatherapy

We've already established that smells are connected to emotions through the limbic system, so aromatherapy can be an effective way to create a pleasant environment. Remember, perfumes and synthetic fragrances can contain toxins, so I encourage you to steer clear of those. However, essential oils can be used in diffusers or other ways to add healing scents to your life.

One study looked at the impact of an essential oil blend (peppermint, basil, and helichrysum) and found that these essential oils might decrease the level of mental exhaustion and moderate burnout.[17]

Here's a round-up of some of my favorite essential oils to diffuse:

- *Lavender* promotes relaxation and sleep; it's also good for relieving stress and easing depression.[18]

- *Peppermint* is good for headaches, digestion, and nausea.[19]

◆ *Eucalyptus* helps your immune system.[20]

◆ *Frankincense,* used in traditional Ayurvedic medicine, can reduce inflammation, improve mood, enhance sleep, and promote gut function.[21]

◆ *Citrus oils,* like lemon, can be uplifting and boost your mood.[22]

Aromatherapy is not expensive, and people generally do well with it. I use an aromatherapy diffuser in my main work and living spaces. I decide which essential oil I would like, based on if I want to feel energized, relaxed, or give my immune system a boost.

Intentionally Color Your Space

Use the information on chromotherapy provided earlier in this chapter to take advantage of how color can impact your mood. Paint is a relatively cheap and easy way to transform your living space; even most rentals will allow you to paint walls in your space, as long as you paint them back before moving out. (Just remember to pick a nontoxic brand!)

Consider using blue in the area where you most often work or use soothing neutral shades of blue, green, and gray to create a calming atmosphere. If bright colors are more your style, try yellow in your kitchen to help you wake up in the morning or violet in your creative space. Leave your blinds open to let in natural light during the day. This will enhance any colors of the room and you'll benefit from seeing the sky out your window.

When it comes to wall art, choose images that make you feel inspired or stoke your creativity. Or you may opt for pictures that are personally significant, like photographs from vacation, images of your family, or works from a local artist that you find especially beautiful. For instance, on one wall, I've displayed photography prints I bought during a favorite vacation I took to the Turks and Caicos Islands; the bright blues of the tropical sea and sky make me happy every time I look at them. Images should invoke good memories and feelings of happiness.

Twenty-Minute Nightly Clean Up

Every night, set aside twenty minutes to pick up clutter, regardless of whether you live alone or with a large family. Researchers in Britain found that cleaning up even for a short period of time can improve mood and counteract depression—not to mention enhance your living space![23] You can tidy up the family room, kitchen, or anywhere there is a mess. In the same way you brush your teeth before bed, this is a quick, easy ritual you can incorporate into your evening routine to make your life more organized.

Never Leave a Room Empty-Handed

Another way to keep your space picked up is to make sure that you never leave a room empty-handed. Whenever you are about to move from one room to another, scan that room for items that need to be put away. Take them with you when you go to another part of the house and put the item in their place.

Ventilate

When the weather is pleasant, open your windows and let fresh air flow into your space. You will feel refreshed by the smell of the air and the circulation from outside. As a result of the air flow, your rooms will be cleared of accumulated toxins emitted by furniture, paint, or carpet. Most people do not realize the importance of allowing fresh air into their homes and either remove their window screens or let them fall apart. Make the most of breezy days by keeping your screens intact, opening your windows, and letting nature flow in. Besides refreshing your space, it will also lift your spirits.

Savor Your Space

"La dolce far niente" is an Italian phrase translated as "the art of doing nothing," referring to the pleasure of being idle. The teaching allows you to stop running yourself ragged and simply enjoy the beauty around you. It is possible to refresh yourself both mentally and emotionally by taking a pause. In other words, doing nothing can be a ritual in itself. Being present allows you to fully experience sounds, smells, and sights wherever you are.

The idea isn't just to be lazy—I don't mean to simply lie on your couch in the dark, scrolling on your phone. This is more about taking a deliberate pause to savor a moment: sit under a tree and watch the clouds as they transform in the breeze. Get on the floor with a baby and watch them discover the world slowly. Take a seat at an outdoor café table and watch the steam rise off your drink as you observe people walking by.

If you deliberately enjoy "la dolce far niente," your body can relax into a more parasympathetic state and you will experience greater joy. Instead of changing the spaces you're in, this ritual aims to simply enjoy them.

HEALTH ON THE INSIDE, SANCTUARY ON THE OUTSIDE

Your living and working space should reflect your personality and be conducive to your physical, mental, and emotional wellbeing. Ideally, the environment in which you live and work should make you feel positive and energized. When you lie down to sleep, it should enable you to get a good night's sleep. When it comes to working, your space should inspire creativity and productivity and nurture a sense of calm when it comes to relaxing. When you invest time in creating a healing space for yourself, you can experience these elements of wellbeing.

Feel the inner calm that comes with a pleasant outer world—and reap the benefits of your pleasant surroundings!

Reflect on Your #CellCare

Using these guiding questions, take a moment to build self-awareness and reflect on your space as a sanctuary in your life:

- Do you feel your home is a place of inspiration? Do you feel relaxed when you are at home?

- Do aspects of your living environment sometimes cause you to feel more stress than ease?

- Does the nature of your space have a positive or negative impact on your relationships with others in your household?

- What are your priorities for your home? With that in mind, what rituals would help create your most ideal home?

Design Your Wellbeing

In the space below, note your thoughts about your main living and working spaces. Where do you see space villains? Where could you incorporate more space heroes? Then, name a ritual you may want to incorporate into your life.

9

EMOTIONAL
EXPLORATION

"Spiritual life is a lot like gardening. We till and cultivate the garden of our heart, planting seeds of presence, openness, and the ability to respect whatever arises. We water each one so the things which are beautiful in us can blossom."

~ JACK KORNFIELD, AUTHOR AND BUDDHIST PRACTITIONER

GUSTAVO WAS A HIGHLY SUCCESSFUL LAWYER, BUT HIS LEGAL career wasn't satisfying anymore. Although his purpose in becoming a lawyer was to promote justice, he questioned whether or not his efforts were serving to help people. Moreover, the stress and long hours were beginning to take a toll on his health. He had symptoms often associated with burnout—fatigue, anxiety, depression, and trouble sleeping—when he came to see me. He was also taking care of his elderly parents, and the stress was compromising him emotionally. Eventually, they passed away, and the grief increased his stress and anxiety significantly, resulting in additional symptoms, including skin rashes and elevated blood pressure.

When Gustavo and I worked together to assess his health habits, we determined they were generally good; however, it was apparent that he needed to make changes to benefit his emotional health. I shared with Gustavo that a person's emotional state could influence physical health. People don't often connect emotions with physical ailments, but emotions have a tremendous impact on our immune functioning, sleep, mental health, and other body systems.

After learning about the effects of his diet on his "happy hormones," Gustavo decided he wanted to adopt a predominantly plant-based diet. He also began to practice yoga and meditation to become more self-aware of his emotional triggers and thoughtfully reflect on his purpose. We incorporated new relaxation techniques into his life, including Epsom salt baths for relaxation and sleep. These de-stressing activities helped mitigate his eczema flare-ups and lower his anxiety. Additionally, we customized his nutrition in order to influence his body's neurotransmitter production and positively regulate his mood.

Gustavo eventually left his career in law to become a meditation teacher. This career change felt personally gratifying and better aligned with what he had come to identify as his purpose: to promote internal peace. In addition, his new community supported his lifestyle changes and enabled him to connect with others in an emotionally rich environment. As a result of making proactive personal and social changes, he became a much happier, healthier person.

INSIGHTS INTO EMOTIONS

Your emotional state has a physiological impact on your body, specifically on your cellular health and immune system—so in other words: on everything![1] Although many people want to write off emotions as unimportant or impediments to success, emotions are critical to your wellbeing. Emotions ultimately determine a person's level of happiness (or unhappiness), which significantly impacts overall satisfaction in life and physical health. Therefore, strengthening your *emotional* health can support your *overall* health and unlock your holistic wellbeing.

Emotional health doesn't mean you're happy all the time—it simply means you have the tools to effectively navigate both positive and negative emotions. To experience life fully, we need to experience many emotions. With that in mind, there are several ways we can describe emotional health:

- ◆ **You are building awareness of your emotions.** As a result, you can increasingly identify what you're feeling and anticipate how those feelings may affect your behavior.

- ◆ You are actively and intentionally **seeking to create a positive, balanced experience** in your life's external events and internal dialogue.

- ◆ **You are open to experiencing a range of emotions.** Rather than bottling them up or avoiding situations where you will be emotionally vulnerable, you make yourself available to feel deeply.

- ◆ **You are learning how to use coping tools** to manage your emotions—both positive and negative—in a constructive way.

By working toward emotional health in these four ways, you're practicing #CellCare for your body and *self-care* for your overall wellbeing. First, by identifying and processing your emotions, you won't bottle them up, resulting in collateral health issues, as seen in Gustavo's story. You're also more likely to mitigate the effects of anxiety and depression on other health issues. Additionally, emotional wellbeing leads to stronger relationships, a healthier self-dialogue, and a clearer sense of purpose—all of which contribute to your body's cellular health and increase overall wellbeing.

In this chapter, we examine the anatomical basis of your emotions, identify factors that contribute to emotional wellbeing, and develop strategies to improve emotional intelligence.

THE ANATOMY OF (EMOTIONAL) WELLBEING

Where do emotions come from? What control do we have—if any—over the way our bodies generate emotions? By understanding how the body produces neurochemicals, we can leverage our biology to constructively process negative emotions and encourage the production of positive emotions.

There are three main aspects of your anatomy that play a significant role in the emotions you end up feeling throughout your day:

◆ **GI System:** Most people are surprised to learn that your gut is responsible for producing a large percentage of your "happy hormones," like serotonin and dopamine. A happy gut helps produce happy emotions.

◆ **Limbic System:** This system includes aspects of the brain like the amygdala, the hippocampus, and the cingulate gyrus. Also known as the seat of your emotional state, the limbic system produces your "fight or flight" stress response and plays a role in emotions like anger or fear.

◆ **Prefrontal Cortex:** This part of your brain, also known as the seat of your executive functioning, governs your rational thinking. This is the part of your anatomy that enables you to choose one thought over another and practice self-control. It's worth noting that the prefrontal cortex is not fully formed until we are adults.

The Conscious Discipline Brain State Model helps us understand the function of the human brain in relation to our behavior, and when we better comprehend how the two work together, we can increase our self-awareness and be more equipped to constructively respond to the needs of the moment. We can learn to consciously manage our thoughts and emotions to arrive at greater emotional wellbeing.

CONSCIOUS DISCIPLINE
BRAIN STATE MODEL

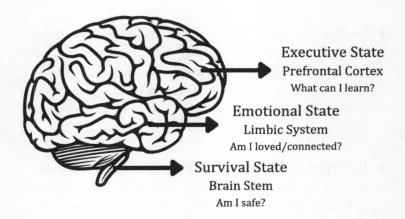

Executive State
Prefrontal Cortex
What can I learn?

Emotional State
Limbic System
Am I loved/connected?

Survival State
Brain Stem
Am I safe?

Most people would say they'd like their bodies to produce more of the happy emotions and less of the stressful ones. Although all emotions can be healthy and warranted in the right time and place, we do have some power over regulating our stress response and ensuring our bodies have the resources they need to produce "happy hormones."

Molecules of Emotion

We've mentioned "happy hormones" throughout this book, but they deserve a spotlight in this chapter. Certain hormones are beneficial for both your body and mood: **serotonin**, **dopamine**, **oxytocin**, and **endorphins**. Your lifestyle choices can facilitate the production of these hormones to help you sleep better, regulate your mood, bond with other people, and take action.

Serotonin regulates your mood and digestion and is essential for getting good sleep and maintaining your circadian rhythm. Few people realize that the gut produces almost *ninety percent* of serotonin. A healthy gut microbiome produces serotonin more efficiently, whereas a damaged gut microbiome struggles to produce this chemical.

> **#CellCare:** Boost your natural **serotonin** levels with nutrition and exercise. Tryptophan-rich foods, such as whole grains, pumpkin seeds, peanuts, soy, pineapple, broccoli, leafy greens, and sesame seeds, can help increase serotonin production. (Tryptophan is a necessary amino acid for the production of serotonin.) Exercise also triggers the release of tryptophan into your blood, which helps generate serotonin. Take your exercise outside—bright sunlight also seems to increase serotonin levels.[2]

Oxytocin, a.k.a. the "cuddle hormone," triggers bonding and compassion responses, helping you form trusted relationships with others. Primarily produced in the brain, oxytocin calms the nervous system and decreases stress. Without sufficient production of the hormone oxytocin, you can feel disconnected from people around you, leading to a feeling of isolation.

#CellCare: You can increase **oxytocin** levels naturally by spending time with loved ones and getting physical touch through cuddling your pet, playing with your child, hugging a friend, or getting a massage. Listening to music[3] and doing yoga[4] can also increase oxytocin levels because they both tend to help us relax.

Dopamine is the feel-good hormone that helps facilitate concentration, motivation, and goal achievement. It's involved in learning and attention and allows you to feel rewarded. When dopamine is low, we don't feel motivated and can feel a general lack of enthusiasm.

Because dopamine contributes to your pleasure response, nice experiences in moderation give you a dopamine hit. That pleasure response motivates you to do that same activity again. (This is why it's hard to eat just one potato chip—your body wants another dopamine hit with each salty crunch!) But if we seek out the dopamine hit over and over again, we come to rely on it—and we need more and more to feel its effects.

In fact, too much dopamine can contribute to addiction. People do many things to get a hit of dopamine that isn't good for them. For example, scrolling social media often gives you a rush of dopamine, but that can become addictive and damaging; too much social media is associated with higher levels of anxiety and depression.[5] The same goes for eating sugar and consuming alcohol or drugs. Indulging in these substances raises the threshold of what you need to get that desired dopamine, and when you don't get enough, it can create emotional lows. Depleted levels of dopamine are also one of the foremost commonalities in people with Parkinson's disease and ADHD.[6]

#CellCare: Dopamine is not a hormone that you want to necessarily "boost" since too much dopamine can contribute to addictive habits. Instead, it's healthier to have *regulated* dopamine levels. To avoid *low* dopamine levels, ensure you're getting enough protein, especially foods with tyrosine and phenylamine; these amino acids help increase dopamine levels. Exercise and probiotic-rich foods can also help in producing dopamine. To avoid too *much* dopamine, practice self-awareness and boundaries. For instance, if you know your social media habits have become addictive, impose a time limit using an app. Also, getting enough sleep is very important for healthy dopamine levels. Insufficient sleep interrupts the dopamine pathway; that, in turn, disrupts your circadian rhythm, resulting in excessive sleepiness.

Endorphins, the neurohormones that are released into your body during exercise, can produce a feeling of exhilaration and play a role in pain relief. Endorphins give you a runner's high or that post-workout feeling of euphoria. Some consider endorphins to be "natural morphine" for the body; they interact with opiate receptors in the brain, similar to how pharmaceuticals alleviate pain. Endorphins help decrease stress, mental distress, and can also provide a feeling of pleasure.

> **#CellCare:** Exercise is your best bet to produce more **endorphins**.[7] Acupuncture also releases endorphins when needles are inserted.[8] Furthermore, endorphins are released during such pleasant experiences as meditation, aromatherapy, performing random acts of kindness,[9] and eating dark chocolate!

The Amygdala's Role in Emotions

The almond-shaped primitive structure in our brain, known as the amygdala, is responsible for our emotional responses such as fear, sadness, and aggression. As we discussed in Chapter Two, the amygdala releases norepinephrine in response to stress, causing electrical impulses to activate our sympathetic nervous system.

The amygdala does more than just trigger our stress response, though—this structure is also what houses our memories of previous experiences and emotions. These play a powerful role in shaping our attitudes for future experiences, triggering us to either anticipate joy or disaster. For example, let's say you went on a family vacation and experienced snorkeling for the first time. The experience was full of happy memories for you—the boat ride was exhilarating, you loved swimming with tropical fish, and the whole experience made for a relaxing day. You would then associate a similar experience positively.

However, imagine that your sibling's experience of the snorkeling trip was completely different. Perhaps she got seasick during the rocky boat ride. When you arrived at the spot to start snorkeling, she slipped going off the ladder and fell into the water without her mask and mouthpiece in place—an embarrassing and painful experience. While snorkeling, her mask kept fogging up and she didn't see a single fish. By the time she returned to the boat, all she cared about was getting back to the hotel room. If you were to suggest going snorkeling again on the next family vacation, your sister would most likely state she had no intentions of going anywhere near a boat or snorkel mask ever again.

We respond strongly to bad experiences because our *negative* memories are stored unequally to protect us from future suffering again, due to their association with painful emotions. In essence, the bad memories take on more "weight" than our positive memories. This protective mechanism can be helpful: our brains want to warn us against repeating experiences that have caused pain in the past. Our negative feelings inform us what we should avoid, protecting us from potential dangers, while our positive emotions inform us what we should pursue.

Sometimes, our amygdala's advice is warranted in signaling experiences that *should* be avoided at all costs in the future. But sometimes, we need to talk our amygdala out of its fear response. In the example of the snorkeling disaster, for instance, you might try to convince your sister that one bad experience shouldn't lead her to swear off snorkeling forever—there's a good chance she'll enjoy it more the next time. And when she does, her amygdala will have the chance to correct its associations with snorkeling. This is where our rational prefrontal cortex plays a role in our emotional health, which we'll discuss more in a moment.

> **#CellCare:** Emotions are created by our experiences. If you dislike an emotion or want to feel a different emotion, cultivating new experiences will be the key to emotional health.

Now, one bad snorkeling trip is an isolated event, but imagine the daily stressors that we experience, which—without our conscious awareness—can commandeer our amygdala. For instance, every time you see, hear, or communicate with your boss, your stress levels spike. The persistent and overactive amygdala activation can negatively impact the function of our prefrontal cortex and hippocampus, leading to poor decision-making and impulsivity. So, even if you don't have a diagnosis of anxiety or PTSD, chronic stress can affect your brain circuitry and adversely influence your wellbeing.

As we discussed in Chapter Two, the brain is like a muscle; the parts of your brain which get the most "exercise" will also be the most robust. That means if you're constantly in a stressful sympathetic state, your amygdala grows larger and produces the stress response more quickly.

On the other hand, if you give your brain and body practice in "resetting" the amygdala, guiding yourself to a parasympathetic state, the neuroplasticity in your brain will strengthen that calming response and keep your amygdala from firing off at a moment's notice.

A daily meditation practice can be a great start to resetting your amygdala and essentially resetting your emotions. For instance, if you know that you are triggered by a certain environmental circumstance, try using a meditation practice to create positive associations, even if that requires you to use mental imagery. Visualization can be a powerful process to activate your frontoparietal control regions to induce a sense of wellbeing. Breathing techniques are yet another way to address emotional states of panic and fear and "reset" your amygdala.

Aside from all of the techniques you may employ, your amygdala may also be influenced by some of the fundamentals of your day. For example, your amygdala may be aggravated by lack of sleep, increased responsibilities, poor self-care, and hormonal imbalances. By seeking to create more balance in these lifestyle areas, you can help regulate the amygdala and prevent it from becoming overactive.

Conflict and stress will inevitably arise in your life, so learning how to cope with challenges is key to building emotional health. In addition to "feeding" your "happy hormones" and learning strategies to reset your amygdala, you have one other powerful anatomical ally in your corner when it comes to building emotional health: your prefrontal cortex.

#CellCare: As a reminder of the parasympathetic protocol we discussed in Chapter Two, there are some simple things you can do to manage stress in your life:

♦ Meditating

♦ Deep breathing

♦ Exercising

♦ Connecting with friends

♦ Participating in activities you enjoy

♦ Listening to music you enjoy

♦ Practicing gratitude

♦ Reflecting on good memories

As you develop a more effective stress management strategy, you may find some of the rituals listed at the end of this chapter helpful to layer on.

Work Out Your Prefrontal Cortex

Your prefrontal cortex is the part of the brain responsible for executive functions such as problem-solving, reasoning, comprehension, creativity, and impulse control. Therefore, being intentional with how you exercise your prefrontal cortex can help counteract the effects of an aggravated amygdala. Again, think about this in terms of working out at the gym: when your amygdala gets the biggest workout, it grows larger and stronger, but if you spend more time deliberately exercising the prefrontal cortex, you help it build gray matter and it becomes the stronger cognitive force. Here are some strategies to do just that:

- **Physical exercise** can increase activity in the prefrontal cortex, especially moderate-intensity exercise.[10] We discussed the power of movement on your cognition in Chapter Five, but it's worth noting here that exercise changes the structure of your brain positively, specifically in the prefrontal cortex and hippocampus. In addition, exercise increases blood flow and production of growth factors such as BDNF, which can cause *neurogenesis*, meaning you're generating new nerve cell growth and increasing your neuroplasticity.

- Ever heard the saying, "**Stepping outside of your comfort zone leads to growth**"? The saying bears up in science. When people try new things, their brains create new neuronal connections that can be strengthened over time—another powerful way to work out your prefrontal cortex. This is precisely what we do when we practice or study something new.

♦ In moments when your amygdala might try to commandeer an otherwise innocuous circumstance with fearful
associations, give your prefrontal cortex the steering
wheel instead. **Prime your prefrontal cortex for
best-case-scenario thinking.** Tell yourself, "I had one
bad experience snorkeling in the past, but I might love
it this time." You can start by noticing your thoughts
without judgment—"I can tell that I'm feeling nervous
and worried, and that's okay"—and being present in the
moment. Then, consider the aspects of the scenario,
and given the facts, make a plan to strategize a best-case
scenario: "I am with great people who I enjoy, I have a
great instructor, and I have good equipment to use. It's
okay if I don't look like a pro, and even if I don't see
the most amazing fish, I can still enjoy being with my
friends in a beautiful place."

♦ If you want to create more gray matter for your prefrontal cortex, you need **sleep, sleep, and more sleep**. So,
put away the electronics, stick to your bedtime, and
indulge in a nighttime ritual. All these steps will help
support your prefrontal cortex, allowing it to be the
stronger cognitive decision-maker for you.

♦ **Reduce highly processed foods** full of sugar, salt,
and artificial additives that can affect your cognition.
Replace them with more fruits and vegetables, which
your brain can use for energy. Many people don't realize that the brain uses energy for thinking and processing emotions, just like your body needs it for physical
activity; nutritious food can help your prefrontal cortex
function at its best.

Now, what do you do with a healthy production of "happy hormones," a subdued amygdala, and a strong prefrontal cortex? You help the prefrontal cortex do its job for your emotional wellbeing by building up emotional intelligence and investing in other key areas that influence emotional health.

> #**CellCare:** Memory resides in the brain, and emotion resides in the body. Our reality is both in our control and under our control.

INCREASING YOUR EMOTIONAL INTELLIGENCE

Imagine going into work and walking on eggshells all day, spending most of your time trying to avoid becoming your boss's next target. Depending on his unpredictable mood, anything is possible—it could be a great day or a day out of a horror film! These are the drawbacks of working with someone who bottles their stress and takes their anger out on other people—often a sign of poor emotional intelligence (EI). EI is our ability to perceive, control, and evaluate emotions. It is a dynamic skill people can build and work at—one that allows us to process our emotions, which plays an important role in our wellbeing.

And what's more, we all *should* be working at this. When developed, EI can provide significant benefits, such as greater life satisfaction, better mental health, improved performance at work, and more rewarding relationships.

Five Emotional Intelligence Skills

Building EI skills will help you be the governor of your emotions, rather than letting your emotions govern *you*. Ever wonder how some people can keep their cool in any situation, while others become overwhelmed and agitated? The individual who practices the five emotional intelligence skills I'm about to discuss may appear calm and collected, even while feeling the same emotions that seem to rattle so many others. EI can lead to greater emotional wellbeing because it can help you stay in a parasympathetic state, ensuring your amygdala stays regulated and your prefrontal cortex remains at the steering wheel.

Here's an example. Let's say that Evita is waiting for her flight at the airport when she finds out her flight is delayed. She has an important meeting to get to and the delay causes her to feel agitated. When Evita approaches the flight attendant to ask for information, the flight attendant can't tell her anything helpful. A person lacking emotional intelligence might be tempted to fly off the handle—but thankfully, Evita has a high level of emotional intelligence and will walk herself through the five emotional intelligence skills: self-awareness, self-regulation, social skills, empathy, and intrinsic motivation. Let's talk about each one.

The first skill to consider is **self-awareness**, or the ability to recognize and monitor your own emotions, but not be controlled by them. Evita might identify her current emotional state and recognize she feels angry and stressed. Then, she introspectively evaluates the emotion, and mindfully realizes that her anger is more connected to fear: she's worried about disappointing the patient she's flying to go see. Now, she has valuable information that allows her to constructively move into the next skill of self-regulation.

You can improve your self-awareness by paying attention to your thoughts and emotions, reflecting on your experiences, and taking feedback as constructive. As discussed in Chapter Two, practicing mindfulness, meditating, and working on a growth mindset also increase self-awareness.

> **#CellCare:** To embrace the full human experience, we must understand and accept that a full range of emotions is part of being an emotionally healthy person. The famous psychologist Robert Plutchik identified eight core emotions that form the foundation for all other emotions:[11]

- Anger

- Fear

- Sadness

- Disgust

- Surprise

- Anticipation

- Trust

- Joy

Even though happiness or joy gives us the most pleasure, the other emotions have an important role to play too. For instance, anger can help motivate us to make needed changes; fear protects us from perceived danger and encourages us to take steps toward safety and health. Part of being an emotionally healthy person involves opening yourself to the full range of emotions, being able to name them (or begin identifying them), and finding strategies to constructively work through them.

Once you've built self-awareness, you're ready to develop **self-regulation**, or the ability to control your emotions. In our illustration, Evita might self-regulate by giving herself a pep-talk: "It's okay that I'm stressed. But I also know that this isn't the end of the world. Getting angry about this isn't going to help me. I can reach out to my patient and I'm sure they'll understand that sometimes, flights just get delayed." Evita processes her emotions by acknowledging that she's stressed and angry—and that those emotions are okay. She adapts to the changes in her schedule by reaching out to her patient. In spite of the uncertainty of her day's plans, she's able to remain calm.

Processing, adapting, and appropriately expressing your feelings: that's what self-regulation looks like. You can help move toward self-regulation by practicing the growth mindset; try to view challenges as opportunities. Understand you have a choice in the way you may respond to a particular situation. This doesn't mean you have to accept something the way it is if you disagree with it. However, it does mean you can manage conflict productively and calmly.

Social skills are one of the most critical aspects of building meaningful relationships. For some, this may come naturally, but for others, this is something that takes intentional practice. People employing effective social skills use nonverbal and verbal cues, along with active listening, to interact and communicate positively with others. We can imagine that, after calming her frustration, Evita approaches the flight attendant with a smile. She begins with a joke to build rapport: "Nice weather we're having, huh?" Then, she proceeds to explain her situation and ask for assistance. She might express gratitude: "I appreciate your help." Establishing a positive dynamic will only help Evita as she navigates the delay.

To improve your social skills, pay attention to your body language and nonverbal cues. For example, crossing your arms and rolling your eyes may be perceived negatively by the other person. These gestures can communicate that you're closed off or dismissive— even if that's not what you intended. An aggressive tone would also be off-putting. On the other hand, you can show a positive attitude with warm facial expressions, open-ended questions, a calm tone of voice, and body language that shows you are open to receive and engage with others—for example, facing a person directly and making eye contact.

Empathy comes next, which is the ability to understand how another person is feeling. For some people, admitting something like, "I can understand how you feel—I've struggled with that too," may appear as a weakness; however, demonstrating empathy is a strength, allowing you to connect with others. In Evita's scenario, she might attempt to connect with the flight attendant by expressing empathy: "I'm sure it's stressful dealing with so many frustrated customers. I have to deal with frustrated patients often too—it sucks!" The flight attendant is likely to feel understood and seen by Evita, setting him up to demonstrate more empathy for Evita's situation as well.

Understanding how someone is feeling and stepping into their shoes is crucial for emotional intelligence. Being empathetic is one way to practice the "golden rule": you're treating others the way that you would want them to treat you in a similar situation. Listening to other people and sharing your feelings is a way to build empathy.

Lastly, **intrinsic motivation** rounds out the skills of emotional intelligence. Instead of seeking external rewards like fame, recognition, or money, someone who is intrinsically motivated is looking for internal rewards, like personal growth, life experiences, or a fulfillment of purpose. Satisfying these inner needs helps a person better align with their purpose and take charge of their own life satisfaction. Rather than depending on circumstances for their fulfillment, they work to improve, grow, and seek their own wellbeing.

In Evita's situation, she might learn from the flight attendant that there is nothing he can do, and no information he can give her—in spite of the pleasant connection that Evita was able to forge. She has one of two choices in that moment: if she is *extrinsically* motivated, she might choose an attitude of victimhood, thinking of all the ways her external circumstances are letting her down: "I'm going to lose this patient; I might lose the commission; my boss will be pissed with me." If she is *intrinsically* motivated, she might look for ways this moment can help her grow: "I'm going to use this time to make my presentation even better." Or she might look for ways to embrace this unexpected life experience: "I'm going to try out one of these nearby restaurants and read my new self-improvement book."

To be clear, Evita might have to be very intentional to practice each one of these skills. Her natural inclination might have been to react strongly and fly off the handle. Any one of us, in emotionally triggering moments, may have to lean hard into our rational prefrontal cortex—reminding ourselves that we can choose to respond constructively, rather than react in a volatile manner.

> **#CellCare:** *Emotional intelligence* can be learned and will increase your resilience. In turn, resilience is linked to better long-term physical and psychological health.

Self-awareness, self-regulation, social skills, empathy, and motivation are the key elements of emotional intelligence, which will help you form strong relationships with other people—including yourself. But why should that be so important in helping you build emotional wellbeing? The fact is—even beyond what's happening in your body and brain—there are other key areas of life, including relationships, that will help you achieve greater emotional health.

YOU ARE MORE THAN YOUR CHEMISTRY

Your hormone production is essential—but it's not everything. There are vital areas outside of your anatomy and hormone production that impact your emotional wellbeing. For example, our beliefs, relationships, resilience, and ultimately the purpose of our lives require our attention to achieve whole-body wellbeing.

For example, **beliefs** inform your ability to love, be compassionate, and forgive. Beliefs are strongly connected to spirituality—the sense that there is something out there beyond yourself, that you belong to a greater whole, and there is more to being human than simply what you experience physically. Research has found that people with spiritual beliefs report better physical health; experience less anxiety, distress, and depression; and tend to practice more health-promoting behaviors.[12] Also described as your ideals or worldview, your beliefs may be demonstrated in your daily behaviors and moral obligations, commonly called values. Your values show up as lifestyle choices and may also inform how you structure your daily practices, such as prayer, meditation, yoga, diet, and how you move your body.

> **#CellCare:** How do you cultivate beliefs if you're not "a spiritual person"? Start by asking yourself probing questions, like "Who am I? Why am I here? What do I value most?" Look for deeper meaning in your life,

such as lessons you may be learning during a hard time. Meditate—be still—and spend time in contemplation to strengthen your values and sense of purpose.

Developing a **robust relational network** is also closely tied to emotional wellbeing. Research shows that a support system improves your health, buffers stress, and allows you to live longer. In addition, "human connection serves to promote health and prevent illness. Conversely, an absence of satisfactory human connection, experienced as loneliness, is detrimental to physical, mental, and social wellbeing."[13]

The author Dan Buettner has compiled a collection of fascinating research about people who live in the world's Blue Zones, which refers to any part of the world where people show remarkable longevity.[14] One of Buettner's most significant discoveries related to relationships: people who live in the Blue Zones have strong community ties. They know their neighbors and other community members, they have friends, and a significant portion of their days are spent connecting with others. It's important to note that, just as I've stressed throughout this book, there was not one single factor that led to the characteristic longevity of the Blue Zones. Everything in our bodies is connected, and Buettner found that people who lived in the Blue Zones also moved their bodies every day and ate nutrient-dense diets. Those factors, plus strong relational ties, help to promote longevity in the world's Blue Zones.

#CellCare: It's important to note that relationships lead to emotional wellbeing only if those relationships are *healthy*. Abusive, manipulative, or toxic relationships can cause far more harm than good. If you sense that a key relationship in your life is purely toxic—in other words, that it couldn't improve with some work—then consider creating a boundary within that relationship to establish a healthy distance. By building healthy self-awareness, you can help yourself recognize when to say NO to others and YES to yourself. This is a meaningful way to care for your emotional wellbeing.

The ability to bounce back after times of struggle is your **resiliency** quotient. So how might resilience inform a person's emotional wellbeing? Imagine that a man goes to the doctor for his annual exam. He learns that he is pre-diabetic. The doctor says if he doesn't do something about it, he'll be on the way to developing full-blown diabetes, requiring lifelong medication. Rather than despairing or resigning himself to a lifetime of medication-dependency, a resilient person would say, "This is not me. I'm athletic and strong. I don't identify with this. I want to heal this condition." He takes the doctor's advice and begins taking steps to resolve the problem. He talks with a nutritionist, changes his eating habits, and ramps up his exercise routine. He wants to *reverse* the condition and seeks every possible way. That's one example of resilience.

Resiliency describes your ability to achieve emotional homeostasis—in other words, the ability to come back to a place of calm. It implies flexibility, a strength, an inner resolve that can allow you to return to equilibrium, even when faced with a significant life challenge. Instead of being sidelined and paralyzed by the unexpected, you have the tools to manage and overcome it. This is not to say that resilient people won't experience difficulties in overcoming, but they can cope with those difficulties and push through.

Finally, a **sense of purpose** outside of yourself is also essential for overall wellbeing. Your purpose is your reason for living. It relates directly to your attitude about making changes in your life, relational health, and spirituality and can considerably impact your physical health. One of the last questions I always ask patients at our initial consultation is, "What is your purpose?" There's usually a pause; people are often surprised by the question. Some people say their purpose is their family; others say it's music, job, or volunteer work. Some people can't identify a clear purpose.

I have observed that my patients who can identify a strong sense of purpose also tend to be the ones who are most willing to make positive changes and seem to heal the fastest. In other words, they have something to live for—and they want to live well. That motivates both their minds and their bodies to heal.

On the other hand, people without a purpose often delay taking the necessary steps toward health. They sometimes go around in circles, ruminating about their health problem. They might think the illness is their fault, like they are being punished in some karmic or cosmic way. These people are *inwardly* focused with no outward focus, which is counterproductive to their healing because they focus on their pain. In the absence of a purpose, the disease can even become a patient's identity. They may even feel like a victim, or like the world is against them. As a result, their illness can take on excessive weight, rather than being a source of motivation—ultimately defining and rewriting who they are.

> **#CellCare:** Japan is ranked second for world life expectancy, and their longevity may be partly due to their focus on purpose. The concept *ikigai* offers guidance in finding the intersection of your passion, mission, and profession, helping you uncover what brings you joy and inspires you to get out of bed every day. The pillars of this philosophy can be used to find strength when times get tough or to plan your life. Start small, live in the moment, release yourself, find harmony and joy in the little things, and most importantly, be present.

A sense of purpose can allow you to look beyond your struggles and focus on how you can make an impact on the world. Being able to contribute and have a purpose in life is invaluable in promoting wellbeing.

RITUALS FOR EMOTIONAL WELLBEING

Given that emotions derive from several different sources and are also influenced by our lifestyles, activities, and mindset, there are many ways we can implement rituals for greater emotional wellbeing.

Connect with Planet Earth

Feeling stressed? Try lying on the ground outside or walking bare-foot in the grass. This process is called *earthing* or *grounding,* and is thought to transfer the Earth's electrons from the ground to your body. This can be done via either direct or indirect contact with the Earth in some of the ways I just mentioned. Alternately—if the weather prevents you from going outside, you can use grounding equipment such as grounding mats or socks, which mimic the electric currents of the Earth. Some research suggests reconnecting with the Earth's electrons can promote physiologic changes and wellbeing.[15] The Earth's energy is important for regulating your body's daily rhythms (such as your sleep–wake cycle) and hormone release, including cortisol. You may also be able to neutralize free radicals involved in your body's immune and inflammatory responses through this influx of free electrons from the Earth, thereby decreasing chronic inflammation.[16] If you experience chronic fatigue, chronic pain, anxiety, depression, sleep disorders, or cardiovascular disease, this may be a technique you want to use.

If you're skeptical, be your own science experiment and give it a try. On the next sunny day or clear night, find a place where you can walk barefoot or lie under the stars. On a scale of one to ten, rate your level of tension and stress before and after the ritual. Using this method, you can deactivate your sympathetic nervous system and shift into a more parasympathetic (i.e., relaxed) emotional state.

Soak Up the Sun

Personally, one of my favorite activities to promote emotional well-being involves letting the sun shine on you. Try and get sunlight exposure at any opportunity for your emotional wellbeing. Sunlight can increase your brain's release of serotonin, the mood-boosting hormone that helps you feel calm and focused. Plus, if you have trouble sleeping and are popping melatonin supplements like M&Ms, consider that your body's natural melatonin production depends on exposure to sunlight. You can improve your mood and sleep by soaking up the sun. In addition, low melatonin levels can affect DNA repair chemicals, ultimately affecting #CellCare.

One of the best ways to boost your happy hormone production is to enjoy the sun first thing in the morning. Consider having your coffee out on the porch or your lunch break in a courtyard. Even getting outside on a gray, rainy day can help you get this needed sunlight—UV rays still penetrate the clouds! Remember that you can also use a sunlight therapy lamp to mimic sunlight. Ultimately, sunlight exposure can boost your levels of serotonin, melatonin, and vitamin D, all of which can impact your emotional wellbeing and your sleep–wake cycle, to name a few. And don't forget, the sunshine can remind you that every day can be a new beginning.

Loving-Kindness Meditation (LKM)

As we've already discussed meditation practices in other chapters, one to consider for enhancing unconditional positive states of kindness and compassion is the Loving-Kindness Meditation. Studies suggest that this practice can strengthen brain areas involved in emotional processing and empathy.[17] In other words, LKM can increase your emotional intelligence! It's a practice that can help you show love to yourself and also help you improve a relationship with someone you're harboring bad feelings against.

For that reason, this type of meditation can improve your relationships and help you cope with anxiety and depression. To try this technique:

- Take a seat in a comfortable position with your eyes closed and muscles relaxed.

- Begin by taking a few deep breaths.

- Imagine yourself in your "happy place"—somewhere where you typically feel emotional wellbeing and inner peace.

- Repeat the following phrases:

  ◇ May I be happy.

  ◇ May I be safe.

  ◇ May I be healthy.

  ◇ May I be peaceful.

- Continue to repeat the phrases, or choose to turn your attention to a loved one:

  ◇ May you be happy.

  ◇ May you be safe.

  ◇ May you be healthy.

  ◇ May you be peaceful.

Continue these phrases to encompass anyone you may want to improve your feelings toward. When your meditation is complete, take a few more deep breaths, then open your eyes and revisit the emotions you generated.

Mood Tracker

To help yourself build self-awareness, try tracking your moods at different intervals throughout the day and week. Note dates, times, and particular events; describe your mood before and after the event, and reflect on your emotions. For example, you might make the following entry:

DATE		
	MORNING	**EVENING**
EVENT	18 holes of golf	See a play with wife
MOOD BEFORE	Energetic, playful, confident, cheerful	Moody, bored, tired
MOOD AFTER	Depleted, grouchy, frustrated, discouraged	Inspired, renewed, engaged
REFLECTION	All the trash talking stresses me out! I need to find new golf buddies.	Should do cultural/ artistic dates like this more often.

This practice can help you build valuable self-awareness and emotional intelligence. It is particularly helpful to identify internal and external triggers that cause fluctuations in your mood. Therefore, once you can identify the triggers, you can utilize different coping mechanisms and determine what does and does not work. Mood trackers, mood journals, or apps can help you correlate and keep track of your emotions. A mood tracker could be the best personal development tool you never knew you needed.

Explore Energy Healing

Albert Szent-Gyorgyi, Nobel Laureate in Medicine, once said, "The cell is a machine driven by energy. It can thus be approached by studying matter, or by studying energy. In every culture and in every medical tradition before ours, healing was accomplished by moving energy." The concept of energy(*qi* or *ojas*) in the body is closely related to emotions. An emotion creates an energetic vibration, which is then felt as thoughts and physical sensations. Ideally, we want to process our emotions and allow that energy to pass through us in a healthy way, freeing us up to experience life with its full range of emotions. However, when we hold on to an emotion, especially a negative one, the energy of that emotion gets stuck and can present itself in physical symptoms. Therefore, from an energetic sense, keeping feelings bottled up can create *dis-ease* and other problems in the body, including pain.

#CellCare: For the mind and body to be healthy, energy has to flow.

Whereas physicians can identify *physical* blockages like cholesterol plaques in an artery, it's difficult to pinpoint and remove *energy* blockages, either mental or emotional. Although energy is invisible to the eye, it is a compilation of your matter, vibrations, and even subatomic particles. Therefore, even though we can't see or comprehend our energy, we can feel it. Using energy healing, which is rooted in 5,000-year-old mind-body healing traditions such as traditional Chinese medicine (TCM) and Ayurveda, we can pursue greater emotional health and alleviate many painful physical symptoms.

How does it work? Energy healing taps into the human bioenergy systems. The meridian system from traditional Chinese medicine, used in acupuncture, is one example of a bioenergy system; the kosha system in Ayurveda is another. These systems map an unseen energy highway that runs through your body. For example, acupuncturists place needles in specific meridian highway points to release blocked energy. By combining mindfulness with the simultaneous activation of specific points on this highway, energy healing can allow us to use ancient whole-body healing practices in the context of modern therapeutics.

People may seek out energy healing practices because of physical discomfort or because they have emotional trauma that feels stuck inside them. Some of the energy healing techniques that help heal physical symptoms include **acupuncture** and **acupressure**. I've also seen patients experience profound emotional healing through the **Emotional Freedom Technique (EFT)** and **reiki**, which focus more on releasing energy tied to emotional trauma. Consider your own emotional and physical state of wellbeing and whether energy healing is a practice that could help you.

Shake It Off—Literally—SHAKE

One of the best ways to get out of a negative emotional state is—as Taylor Swift would say—to shake it off, physically moving your way out of it. If you are sitting, stand up. If you are inside, go outside. You need to move the energy through you so that it doesn't get stuck inside you. And if it still feels stuck, then go ahead and shake it off. I mean that literally—shake your body!

Shaking can help regulate the nervous system and release tension and trauma from the body by burning excess adrenaline and releasing muscle tension. I recall one of my integrative professors starting a class with us standing up and just shaking our bodies to the beat of tribal drums. Although this initially felt strange to me, I often remember the feeling it left in my body and how my tenseness dissipated within a few minutes. She called it shaking.

How exactly does it work? Shaking uses two opposing functions to regulate the body's autonomic nervous system. The mere act sends a signal to your parasympathetic nervous system and signals it to relax. The end result: shaking eases an overstimulated nervous system.

Ready to try it? Stand with your feet hip-width apart, drop your shoulders, and begin shaking. Feel the bounce through your knees and allow the vibration to spread to your arms, neck, and shoulders. At the same time, consider what your body feels like before doing this and how it feels after doing this.

Labyrinth Meditation

Labyrinths are winding paths representing a journey to a predetermined destination while performing a walking meditation from the edges to the center. Around the world, these structures are known for bringing peace and harmony to the mind, calming the nervous system, and restoring the body's natural spirit. While there is no right or wrong way to traverse a labyrinth, it's possible to gain guidance using the Three Rs.

- ♦ Release: As you enter, let go of whatever you wish to leave behind.

- ♦ Receive: Upon reaching the center, receive whatever you are ready to receive.

- ♦ Return: Leave the same way you arrived, and carry with you what you have received.

Walking a labyrinth can promote your mental, physical, and spiritual wellbeing. You can find a local path at labyrinthlocator.com or create one for your use if you have the space.

Find Your Inner Artist

Many artistic activities, including painting, dancing, drawing, and even writing, can lower stress levels and provide mental calmness. Making art can also allow you to process your emotions and express yourself without using words. The idea is that creative expression can foster healing and mental wellbeing.[18]

You might be thinking, "I'm not creative. I can't draw or paint—and what exactly does this have to do with my emotional wellbeing, anyways?" First of all, making art—even bad art—can be great for your emotional health. One neuroscience research study found that visual art—like sculpting, drawing, or painting—promotes health, wellness, and improves our ability to respond to stress.[19] Newer research in the field of neuroaesthetics—which uses brain wave technology and biofeedback to gather scientific evidence on how we respond to art—suggests that "creating art can reduce cortisol (your body's main stress hormone) and induce a positive mental state."[20] That is to say, finding your inner artist may be an effective way to manage your mental and emotional wellbeing.

And no one's asking you to be Picasso. The beauty of finding your inner artist is to provide relaxation from the day-to-day stressful situations—regardless of whether or not your artistic expressions are anything to write home about. There are many easy and fun ways you can start incorporating art into your life. Consider a local paint night with the girls or a woodworking class to build a sign for your front porch. Even an evening dance party with your kids is an opportunity for artistic expression—and bonding!

Set Personal Boundaries

Most of us feel an inherent need to be liked, to appear kind and not let others down. Because of this, some people may not be the best at saying no to others and yes to themselves. That's where personal boundaries can play a key role in your emotional wellbeing.

Setting personal boundaries can help you gain a sense of control over how you live your life and spend your time, which can be beneficial for you and the people around you. For example, you might commit to getting a workout in the morning—even though it means time away from your kids—because you know it will help you be a better parent for the rest of the day. These boundaries can also help you clarify your beliefs and values, gain a greater sense of identity, avoid burnout, and increase your emotional wellbeing. You might feel reluctant to disappoint someone who has asked you to do something you don't have time for. However, rather than assuming someone will be upset with you, simply explain your situation and ask the person how they feel to avoid misunderstandings.

Next, make your boundaries non-negotiables. If you always compromise and do not follow your boundaries, you may create unnecessary emotional turmoil. Learn to take time to collect your thoughts and communicate them when sharing your feelings with someone—the EI skills can help with this.

If someone does not respect your boundaries, consider moving on from this relationship for your emotional wellbeing. Boundary setting is an essential aspect of self-care and #CellCare.

Digital Detox

You may or may not realize it, but our social media–focused culture significantly impacts our emotional wellbeing. There's a good side and a bad side to your virtual connections. You may think you feel more connected when you see what is going on social media. Still, the reality is it creates feelings of inadequacy, dissatisfaction, and isolation.[21] Interactions with technology cannot compare to the companionship of a human being another person. We are social creatures, and lack of real connectivity can lead to irritability, stress, and depression.

How can you use social media positively? Social media can be a great way to communicate with friends and family worldwide, find new communities, and join worthwhile causes. When used in moderation, social media can add to your life.

However, if you sense that you're constantly feeling "the grass is greener on the other side" as you scroll through your friends' idyllic posts, social media might be harming more than helping. You may compare yourself to others, leading to dissatisfaction with your own life and exacerbating anxiety.

How do you know if you need a digital detox? Here are a few things to consider:

- ◆ Do you find yourself distracted at work and school and obsessively checking your phone for likes and follows?

- ◆ Do you spend more time on social media than with real people?

- ◆ Is social media the first thing you check in the morning and the last thing you check before you go to bed?

- ◆ Do you feel more lonely, irritable, or anxious after using social media?

If you answered yes to any of these, consider this a reality check for an intentional digital detox (the only kind of detox I endorse for your #CellCare). Follow these steps to get a grip on your screen time:

◆ Turn off push notifications—the alerts that tell you what is going on, which can be highly distracting.

◆ Put your phone away during certain times—for example, when eating a meal, when playing with your kids, when walking in nature—be present in what you are doing. Consider using these moments as an opportunity to practice mindfulness instead.

◆ Make your bedroom a tech-free zone. This will not only help you sleep better but can also create greater intimacy in the bedroom.

◆ Designate a daily tech-free hour—this is a great activity to do with the family. Taking a deliberate break from your devices can help inspire your creativity and allow your mind to be stimulated in another way.

◆ Declutter your phone—just as your desktop gets clogged up with unnecessary documents, your phone may have apps on there that no longer serve a purpose. Once at least every quarter, set aside time to declutter what's there and only keep what you use.

MIND, HEART, SOUL

I have spent nearly half of my life studying the human body. I find it fascinating! But I find it equally fascinating that our health is so profoundly affected by forces we cannot see under a microscope: our emotions and energies. I encourage you to cultivate greater emotional wellbeing by using science and then going beyond what science can prove. You can significantly increase your happiness by noting what affects your "happy hormones." The expansion of your emotional intelligence, the development of stronger relationships, the embrace of spiritual practices, the identification of a purpose, and the examination of your energy flow can all contribute to your emotional wellbeing. As a result of these powerful and mysterious elements, wellbeing will be enhanced even further.

Reflect on Your #CellCare

Using these guiding questions, take a moment to build self-awareness and reflect on your emotional wellbeing:

- ♦ What is your perspective on allowing yourself to feel both positive and negative emotions? Do you believe that experiencing the full range of emotions is part of living a meaningful, fulfilling life?

- ♦ How are you supporting your "happy hormones"? Between the amygdala and the prefrontal cortex, what tends to govern your emotions?

- ♦ Of the five emotional intelligence skills, where do you feel you excel? Which skill would you like to develop more?

- ♦ Do you feel your purpose supports your beliefs and your relationships? Reflect on your resiliency.

♦ Do you tend to bottle up your emotions, or express them freely? Is it possible you're experiencing the effects—either physically or emotionally—of an energy blockage?

DESIGN YOUR WELLBEING

In the space below, note your thoughts about your emotional wellbeing. Then, name a ritual you may want to incorporate into your life.

10

LEVELING UP

"I believe that you can, by taking some simple and inexpensive measures, lead a longer life and extend your years of wellbeing. My most important recommendation is that you take vitamins every day in optimum amounts to supplement the vitamins that you receive in your food."

~ LINUS PAULING, AMERICAN CHEMIST

WHEN I FIRST MET GABRIELLE, I COULD TELL RIGHT AWAY that she was incredibly proactive about her health. She was eager to do a "functional body audit" to gather as much data as possible about her cellular health. While waiting for our follow-up appointment, she reviewed her lab results and decided to take action on her perceived deficits.

Gabrielle went to her local drug store, and—by studying her lab paperwork—began to fill up her basket with supplements. When I next spoke with her, she shared this development proudly and was

THE ANATOMY OF WELLBEING

surprised when I expressed concern. I could see that she was looking at her supplement needs as a simple math equation: she was
deficient in X, therefore, she needed to take supplement X. I tried
to explain that the human body is a bit more complex than that.

First, dosages and brands matter for efficacy, I explained. Secondly,
people absorb both food and supplements differently, depending on how their bodies work. Just because a supplement says
it provides "250% of DV," that doesn't mean your body actually
absorbs 250 percent. In order to accurately assess her supplement
needs, we needed to evaluate both her body's ability to absorb
nutrients and her dietary intake. In other words, the time, money,
and effort she had put into sorting out her own supplementation
may not have led to the results she was after. Gabrielle was well
informed about her symptoms—but still needed the guidance of
an integrative physician to fully understand how to meet her own
unique requirements.

Her digestion was improved and she was shown how to get the
most vitamins and minerals she needed from a balanced, nutrient-rich diet. We then added targeted supplements to fill in the
gaps, including reviewing what she had purchased. Some of them
were of poor quality, contained unhealthy "fillers," or were unnecessary. Those went into "the supplement graveyard": the trash can
next to my desk.

WHAT YOU NEED TO KNOW
ABOUT SUPPLEMENTS

Supplements seem to offer a quick, easy fix to solving your health
problems. Although most of us would benefit from some *targeted*

supplementation to address genuine deficiencies, there is no one-size-fits-all. Supplements are not a silver bullet; there's no shortcut to being healthy. However, the supplement industry—worth more than $120 billion—wants to capitalize on people's desire to be healthier by making you think a pill can solve your problems. Unfortunately, these marketing efforts lead people like Gabrielle astray.

> **#CellCare:** There is no shortcut to being healthy. A targeted and tailored strategy of supplementation with monitoring labs can generate positive results, whereas a generalized, nonspecific approach can have the opposite effect.

Before we get into specifics about supplements, let's talk about what they are. A dietary supplement is defined as a product taken by mouth that contains an ingredient (or ingredients) intended to *add to the nutrients you're getting through your diet.* These ingredients include vitamins, minerals, herbs, botanicals, amino acids, and metabolites. (We haven't talked about metabolites yet; they help facilitate the chemical reactions your body needs to function well.) Supplements come in many forms, such as capsules, gels, liquids, powders, and tablets. They're also trendy—but they should be used with caution.

I like to think of supplements as decorations for your body, just as you might put on a Christmas tree. Ideally, when it's time to decorate for the holidays, you're going to start with a healthy, green, full tree. However, if a Christmas tree is old, brown, and sickly in appearance, putting more decorations on top won't make the tree look much better—you want to put ornaments on a healthy and flourishing tree. Therefore, supplementation should be used *in addition to* all the other practices I've discussed in this book that will revitalize your body and help you maintain good health. Of course, to be that healthy green Christmas tree, you need wholesome nutrition, adequate rest, purposeful exercise, and so on. Those are the factors that will help your body flourish. *Then* it's time to add the supplements on top, to *fill in the gaps.*

There's a reason this chapter on supplements comes last: ideally, you will address the other areas of your lifestyle before turning to this one. Supplements are not intended to replace exercise or healthy eating habits; they should complement your nutrition when you are unable to absorb certain nutrients, have a nutritional deficiency for reasons beyond your control, or have symptoms that require treatment.

The Back Story of Supplements

When you understand how supplements are regulated in this country, you might develop a healthy skepticism about the industry. In 1994, Congress passed a new law called the Dietary Supplement Health and Education Act (DSHEA), which created new regulations for the safety and labeling of supplements. Under the DSHEA, a supplement company is responsible for determining if a supplement, its manufacturers, and its distributors are safe and that any representations or claims are substantiated by adequate evidence.

This means dietary supplements *do not need FDA approval* before they are marketed, except in the case of a new dietary ingredient where a pre-market review of safety data and other information is required by law. In addition, a supplement company does not have to provide the FDA with any evidence of efficacy.

Did you catch that? Unlike pharmaceuticals, which go through several phases of research and testing, a supplement being marketed to you as a "silver bullet cure-all" may not have Phase 2 or 3 trials to determine their safety or effectiveness. This is why you'll see a disclaimer on supplements stating the FDA does not evaluate them, and the product is not intended to diagnose, treat, cure, or prevent any disease. This disclaimer distinguishes supplements from medications.

Unfortunately, this lack of regulation can confuse consumers. Many supplements *have* been studied and shown to be *beneficial*, but it's tough for consumers to find the good ones amongst the pile of snake oil supplements with no proven efficacy. As an example, one patient showed me collagen gummy bears for her hair, skin, and nails—but the first two ingredients were sugars that worked directly *against* her skin improvement goals. Due to these lax regulations, good marketing can easily sway consumers, regardless of whether a supplement is targeted to meet their nutritional needs.

> **#CellCare:** Speaking of collagen, let's talk about this trendy supplement, which promises to help with anti-aging. Our bodies cannot readily absorb collagen from topical creams or ingestible powders; however, by eating plant-based foods (such as seeds, lentils, chickpeas, and beans), we can absorb its building

blocks. Diets rich in vitamin C, from citrus fruits and bell peppers, proline, from cabbage, mushrooms, and asparagus, and copper and zinc, from cashews, sesame seeds, and lentils, are necessary for collagen production. If you want to work on your wrinkles, try eating some of the foods I just listed. Rather than using collagen supplements as an anti-aging magic trick, give your body nourishing food, hydration, and sleep. You'll keep feeling and looking youthful with these lifestyle practices.

When taking supplements, it's imperative to understand how they may interact with your other medications and vitamins, along with your diet. A good physician familiar with supplements and botanicals will look for those indications based on your bloodwork and other physiological data.

Can Supplements Cause Harm?

You might be wondering, "Is it such a big deal if I'm taking the wrong vitamins? They're still more likely to help than harm, right?"

Wrong!

Supplements can cause harm when taken in mega-doses or not taken appropriately, and there can be side effects when combined with certain medications. Here are some examples:

- Too much B6 (found in many multivitamins) can cause nerve issues and/or liver damage.

- Excess selenium (taken for thyroid problems) can cause hair loss, fatigue, and cause GI issues.

- Taking too much zinc or vitamin C (taken for immune health) can create digestive problems such as diarrhea or stomach cramps, whereas your body would benefit much more from simply eating oranges, berries, or red peppers.

- Fat soluble vitamins, such as D, E, A, and K (taken for a variety of reasons) are not excreted through the urine, like vitamins C or B. Instead, they are stored in the body tissues and can be potentially harmful. For example, mega-doses of vitamin A can cause nausea, loss of bone density, and headaches. Excess vitamin D can cause irregular heartbeats.

- Supplements can also interact with medications that you might be taking in unexpected and harmful ways.

Remember, your body is *made* to collect and absorb these necessary ingredients from your food. Your cells will be happier with vitamin C from an orange than a pill.

Many supplements aren't so much harmful as they are useless. For instance, gummy vitamins have got to go. I place these vitamins in a broad, general category because most don't contain the necessary nutrients to counteract the sugars that make them so tasty. While some are okay, many vitamins and supplements may not provide optimal levels. They're also not likely to be tailored to your specific health concerns, which you'll probably need some help to assess.

> **#CellCare:** Many people spend years taking their own assortment of supplements because they don't want to take the time to go see a doctor trained in supplements. However, these years can easily be wasted if you're inadvertently giving your body supplements it doesn't need or taxing it by taking vitamins in excess. You'll need around two to three appointments with a doctor trained in this area in order to get a tailored, clear picture of your body's supplement needs. Look for an integrative or functional doctor, trained in identifying vitamin and mineral deficiencies. It's a short-term investment of your time that will pay off enormously in the long run.

Can you take *any* supplements confidently, before seeing a doctor? At a minimum, I recommend people start with a quality multivitamin, vitamin D, and an omega-3 supplement. From there, you're going to want to get tailored recommendations. I recommend a blood test to determine your body's unique deficiencies. For example, your need for vitamin D can range, but you won't know your particular needs unless you have bloodwork done first.

However, for everyone who isn't jumping on the phone with a functional medicine doctor, you can still improve your own efforts at supplementation by developing a better understanding of what your body needs. Rather than just taking a pill that's been marketed well, start with an understanding of what your cells need to function optimally.

#CellCare: Some general tips to supplement your body well:

- Look for seals of approval, such as the USP seal or the NSF seal—these indicate the supplements have been tested for safety and efficacy.

- Consider a separate supplement when your multivitamin doesn't have your recommended daily value.

- Many of the plant compounds I recommend in this chapter can be taken safely in small doses with your food—for example, turmeric or rosemary. However, if you want a therapeutic level to address a specific disease or symptom, you may require these in supplement form; in that case, I strongly recommend you consult an integrative or functional medicine physician to ensure proper dosage.

- Many supplements are meant to be taken for a *finite* amount of time, but not indefinitely. With aging, your body changes, and your nutritional needs change, which means that your supplement needs may also change.

♦ It's always best to get the lion's share of your nutrients through your food. This is what the body is built to do, and food provides the body with the nutrients it needs.

Targeted Supplementation:
What *Does* Your Body Need?

With all that said, I want to clarify that I'm definitely not anti-supplementation. Personally, I take supplements myself, and all my patients take them, but I promote what I call *targeted supplementation*. This means taking supplements for a specific purpose or addressing a legitimate need for your body. With this targeted supplementation, I use measurable factors, review for cross-reactivity, and adjust dosing, just as you would for a medication.

The two major categories of supplements are **vitamins** and **minerals**. In Chapter Three, you learned that vitamins are substances found in our food that our bodies need to develop and function properly. Minerals are inorganic compounds found in soil and water; they include calcium, magnesium, copper, zinc, iron, selenium, and iodine. However, a few aspects of our modern world have led to decreases in the nutrient content in our food.

First, our over-farmed soil and water are becoming depleted of these minerals, which has changed the nature of our food supply. As a result, you may have certain vitamin and mineral deficiencies that would benefit from supplementation.

Moreover, the distance produce has to travel before reaching its destination influences its nutrient content. For instance, if someone in Minnesota wants to eat strawberries in January, they probably come from a warmer climate, like California. Since many days will pass between the time the strawberry is picked and the time it is consumed, nutrients can be lost when food travels long distances. This is because foods "respirate" as soon as they're picked, losing flavor and nutrients with each passing day. (Locally sourced foods are typically tastier, fresher, and more nutrient-dense.) Secondly, foods go through an enzyme process after getting picked, further causing nutrient loss. Take the example of fruits and vegetables that turn brown as they age due to an enzymatic process that begins to break them down. Likewise, a food's nutrient quality will be affected by their ripeness; a green, unripe banana will be high in resistant starch, low in sugar, and lower in antioxidants, whereas a ripe banana will have less starch, more sugar (higher glycemic index), and higher antioxidants.

Vendors have found creative ways to get around the problem of produce items losing their freshness, but their "solutions"—namely, preservatives—are not great for our health either. Some foods may undergo treatment to support their "freshness." Do you know what makes your grocery store apples look so shiny? This is a wax sprayed on apples to prevent moisture from escaping when it needs to travel long distances. But it's not just apples—sometimes cucumbers, peppers, tomatoes, and even citrus fruits will have it.

Some coatings are natural wax, whereas others are synthetic petro-leum-based; either way, our body cannot digest or break down the wax. You can help remove the wax by using a fifty-fifty mixture of vinegar and water or removing the skin (which also depletes some nutrients). And baby carrots may be cute and tasty, but they are washed in chlorine (another preservative) before packaging. You are better off eating adult carrots (you know, the ones that haven't been drenched in chlorine to kill bacteria and preserve them). I recommend getting locally grown and sourced food whenever possible to avoid preservatives.

We discussed your body's vitamin and mineral needs in Chapter Three. As a reminder, here are some of the essential vitamins and minerals your body needs for cellular health.

When it comes to supplementation, we need to look at common deficiencies in these categories. Overall, some of the most common deficiencies worldwide are magnesium, vitamin D, calcium, zinc, vitamin B12, vitamin A, iodine, and iron. Nevertheless, before you start supplementing yourself, remember that all your levels should be checked thoroughly with blood work.

You can prevent vitamin deficiencies by—any guesses? Eating a predominantly nutrient-dense whole-foods diet—ideally, organic and locally sourced—along with avoiding processed foods, sugar, and refined carbs.

When to Take Supplements

It's not just essential to consider *what* supplements to take—you also want to pay attention to *when* you take them.

VITAMINS FOR CELLULAR HEALTH

VITAMIN B1
Supports energy production, nerve function, and digestion
(Brazil nuts, lentils, spinach)

VITAMIN B2
Key in antioxidant function, energy production, detoxification, and vitamin activation
(almonds, broccoli, asparagus, mushrooms)

VITAMIN B3
Involved in DNA repair, cell differentiation, fatty acid, and cholesterol synthesis
(lentils, seeds, peanuts)

VITAMIN B6
Important for synthesis of neurotransmitters, heme, and red blood cells
(soybean, nuts, seeds, carrots)

VITAMIN B7
Involved in DNA replication, fatty acid synthesis, and immune health
(avocado, raspberries, cauliflower)

VITAMIN B9
Involved in cell renewal, DNA synthesis, and red blood cell production
(beans, legumes, leafy green vegetables)

VITAMIN B12
Key in maintenance of nerve tissue and red blood cell production
(chlorella, nutritional yeast, supplement)

VITAMIN A
Involved in gene expression, cell growth, antioxidant and immune function, and eye and skin health
(kale, pumpkin, sweet potato)

VITAMIN C
Important antioxidant involved in cholesterol metabolism and synthesis of collagen, white bloods cells, and antibodies
(strawberries, oranges, tomato, broccoli)

VITAMIN D
Important for bone health, cardiac function, immune health, body weight maintenance, and prevention of cancer
(sunshine, supplements, mushrooms, fortified non-dairy milk)

VITAMIN E
Toxin elimination, cell protection, and immune function
(sunflower seeds, almonds, collard greens, spinach,)

VITAMIN K
Involved in protein synthesis for blood clotting and building bones
(cabbage, kale, kiwi, spinach)

NOTE
All B vitamins help cells convert food into energy (ATP) and metabolize fats and protein

MINERALS FOR CELLULAR HEALTH

MANGANESE
Supports thyroid function, muscle
reflexes, and the nervous system
(dark leafy green vegetables,
legumes, nuts)

COPPER
Aids in fighting infections and
supports lung and kidney
function
(beans, nuts, dark leafy green
vegetables, prunes, cocoa)

CHROMIUM
Affects insulin sensitivity
and macronutrient
metabolism
(cabbage, romaine
lettuce, celery, onions)

IODINE
Assists in thyroid hormone
production and regulating
metabolism
(seaweed, soybean, watercress)

IRON
Carries oxygen from the lungs to
the rest of your body and is used to
make hemoglobin for red blood
cells
(dark leafy green vegetables, beans,
legumes, nuts, seeds)

CALCIUM
Supports healthy bones and teeth,
blood clotting, normal heart rhythms
and nerve function
(soybean, bok choy, kale, watercress,
chickpeas)

ZINC
Supports a healthy immune
system, DNA synthesis, gene
expression, and growth of cells;
repairs damaged tissue and
decreases inflammation
(nuts, seeds, legumes, soybean,
oats)

POTASSIUM
Functions as an
electrolyte to maintain
normal fluid levels inside
cells and regulates nerve
signals and muscle
contractions
(Swiss chard, lentils,
dried apricots and figs,
squash, avocado)

PHOSPHORUS
Important for production of
genetic material (DNA and
RNA), helps balance other
vitamins and minerals, and
needed for growth and repair
of all tissues and cells
(peanuts, cashews, walnuts,
quinoa, soybean,

MAGNESIUM
Involved in more than 300
chemical reactions in the body;
supporting muscle and nerve
function, energy production,
cardiovascular health, bone health,
sleep health, and mental health
(pumpkin seeds, pistachios,
oatmeal, cocoa)

You will want to take certain supplements with food. For example, the fat-soluble vitamins—D, E, A, and K—are best taken with fatty food, like avocados or a handful of nuts, because it allows your body to better absorb the vitamin.

If you take a supplement that contains any B vitamins, don't take it at night because it will keep you wired. Instead, take them in the morning; they'll help you wake up and provide you with a boost of energy. People sometimes take these B supplements with their dinner, and then wonder why they feel wide awake and can't sleep. (*Psst,* it was your B vitamins!)

Also, if you are on any medications, you definitely want to consult with your doctor for appropriate timing and efficacy.

FUEL YOUR BODY

So, what are some of the best ways to get the nutrients your body needs *before* turning to supplements? The answer, as usual, starts with what you eat.

Superfoods

As a relatively new term, "superfoods" refer to foods with maximum nutritional benefits, packed with vitamins, minerals, and antioxidants. Another way to define a superfood is "nutrient-dense and calorie-poor"—in other words, you get a huge amount of nutrients for a comparatively small amount of calories. The following are some top contenders that are packed with nutrition:

♦ **Berries:** Berries contain nineteen amino acids and many antioxidants. As a reminder, antioxidants neutralize free radicals in the body, which are substances that cause a significant amount of cellular damage and are involved in the aging process. Try blueberries, goji berries, acai, raspberries, and cranberries. *Goji berries* are especially beneficial because they contain high amounts of vitamin C, vitamin E, and flavonoids. Vitamin C can help kidney and liver health and support the immune system. You can find goji berries in the dried fruits section of most grocery stores—try eating a handful rather than taking a vitamin C supplement.

♦ **Soy:** This superfood is controversial because it's one of eight major food allergens. However, if you're not allergic to soy, this food provides many nutritional benefits. Soy contains isoflavone, which can help lower bad cholesterol, prevent bone loss during menopause, and age-related memory loss. Many women are susceptible to bone loss because the Western pattern diet (a.k.a. the SAD) doesn't often include soy, making this a particularly good food for that demographic. Soy is also protective against some cancers. When buying soy, make sure you're purchasing non-GMO, organic soy. The best sources are tofu, edamame, and soy milk.

♦ **Green tea:** Chock full of antioxidants, green tea also has anti-inflammatory[1] and anticarcinogenic properties.[2] Many studies show it has overall health benefits that stem from its unique chemicals, L-theanine and EGCG. L-theanine promotes relaxation and facilitates sleep; it also increases GABA, serotonin, and dopamine. EGCG is a powerful antioxidant that protects from cellular damage. In addition, a study conducted with students revealed that green and white tea could reduce stress levels.[3] Green tea is an excellent alternative to coffee, and—since it can suppress inflammation—it's especially beneficial for people who experience joint pain.

♦ **Dark leafy greens:** Kale, spinach, and Swiss chard are examples of dark greens high in vitamins C, E, K, and B. They're also high in magnesium, potassium, calcium, and iron. Talk about a superfood! When making a salad, use dark leafy greens rather than romaine or iceberg because these light-colored lettuces don't pack quite the nutritional powerhouse.

♦ **Cruciferous vegetables:** Broccoli, broccoli sprouts, bok choy, and cabbage contain a sulfur-rich component called *sulforaphane*, which has potent anti-inflammatory and antioxidant properties. Sulforaphane is also suitable for creating a healthy gut microbiome, and it has potential anti-cancer benefits.

♦ **Avocados:** This vitamin-rich food is high in fiber, low in carbs, and contains the healthy monosaturated fats your body needs to decrease inflammation and heart disease. Avocados can help with appetite regulation and weight loss. People often go on low-fat diets because they think fat will cause weight gain when, as we've discussed, they need to eat the *right* fats, like avocados, instead. Healthy fats can satisfy your cravings, feed your brain and body, and prevent you from reaching for a snack. A baby avocado a day will keep your brain happy.

♦ **Turmeric:** This spice contains an active compound called curcumin, which has potent antioxidant and anti-inflammatory effects.[4] However, people sometimes overestimate the effectiveness of the culinary form of turmeric to reduce their inflammation. That's because the active compound in the spice that produces its anti-inflammatory effects, curcumin, is quite low. In order to get a truly therapeutic anti-inflammatory effect, you may need to supplement turmeric with piperine to help its absorption and effectiveness. Either way, turmeric is an easily accessible and potent spice with beneficial properties. It may be a suitable supplement for people who suffer from chronic low grade levels of inflammation, as seen in cancer, Alzheimer's and heart disease. Curcumin can also increase BDNF;[5] remember, that's the protein important for memory and learning. Likewise, it has proven more effective than anti-inflammatory drugs for rheumatoid arthritis.[6]

♦ **Asian mushrooms:** Ugrading your palate to shiitake, maitake, enoki, oyster, and lion's mane has a host of health benefits. For example, lion's mane contains *hericenones*, which help stimulate the growth of brain cells, while shiitake contains *eritadenine*—a compound that can help reduce cholesterol—and *beta-glucans* that reduce inflammation.

♦ **Tart cherries:** Cherries have a compound, melatonin, that helps promote better sleep, so people with sleep issues can benefit from drinking cherry juice regularly.[7] They're also good for joint pain and weight loss, so I suggest getting cherries whenever they are in season.

#CellCare: For a tasty treat that will help you sleep well, try this sleep-inducing trio. In the evening, prepare a beverage of tart cherries, pistachios, and almond milk. Tart cherries, as already mentioned, are a great source of melatonin. Pistachios contain melatonin, B6, and magnesium, which can help you sleep. Lastly, almonds are a natural source of tryptophan, which your body needs to sleep well

Ingredients:

- ¼ cup frozen cherries

- ¼ cup shelled pistachios

- 1 cup almond milk

Directions:

In a high-speed blender, combine all three ingredients, blend until smooth, and enjoy right away.

One of my favorite superfoods doesn't come from a farm—it comes from the ocean. There are two types of algae that are also considered superfoods: spirulina and chlorella.

- **Spirulina:** This blue-green microalga produces energy from sunlight. Although tiny, a single tablespoon of this algae contains four grams of protein—comparable to the protein in eggs. Spirulina is high in B vitamins, copper, calcium, and iron. In addition to lowering cholesterol[8] and blood pressure,[9] it is also a powerful antioxidant[10] and anti-inflammatory. Spirulina is easy to add to your smoothies or into some homemade energy bites. For expectant mothers, athletes, or anyone looking to support their immune system, spirulina is an ideal ingredient for your snacks.

- **Chlorella:** This microalga helps the body bind to heavy metals, enabling the body to eliminate heavy metal toxins.[11] It also supports the immune system,[12] is easy on the digestive tract, can boost energy, and reduce morning stiffness and achiness. As an excellent source of vitamin B12, it suitable for vegans. In addition, it may help lower cholesterol and blood pressure levels.[13] Furthermore, chlorella is composed of fifty percent protein and is rich in fiber and vitamin C.

These superfoods can do wonders for your nutritional intake before you ever reach for a bottle of supplements. However, there are two more plant-based fuel categories worth learning about: botanicals and adaptogens.

BOTANICALS

Before pharmaceuticals became widespread in the twentieth century, most healing was done using medicinal plants. These plants haven't stopped being helpful—and in fact, we now know more about their medicinal properties than ever before. These remarkable healing plants form the category of botanicals.

Botanicals are plants (or parts of plants, such as the root or the flower) valued for their therapeutic or medicinal properties. They can even be valued for their flavors and scents, and we can use botanicals to improve or maintain health. Sometimes, they're called *phytonutrients*, as I referred to them in Chapter Four, or "plant medicine." Botanicals can also be used as a preventative measure in addition to treating illness. These medicinal plants have several categories, and some we will discuss include adaptogens, cognitive-support botanicals, and nervines.

Adaptogens

An adaptogen is an herb that is specifically useful for modulating the stress response. It creates balance in the hypothalamus and the pituitary and adrenal glands, meaning that if your stress levels are high, adaptogens can help bring them back down to homeostasis. But also, if you're feeling "blah" on the lower end, adaptogens can help raise your "feel good" hormones, helping to elevate your mood. In other words, adaptogens help balance you out, wherever you're at on the stress spectrum. You can think of them as a "plant-based hack" against the stress response. One study found that adaptogens promote health and general wellbeing, also finding they could modulate and protect the central nervous system, have an anti-depressive effect, and fight fatigue.[14] There's a lot this category of botanicals can do for your mood!

When taking adaptogens, the goal is to determine which ones you need and then find your "sweet spot." Adaptogens aren't expensive, but make sure that whatever adaptogens you purchase are organically grown so they don't contain pesticides or other chemicals. I also recommend researching adaptogen brands and going with a reliable manufacturer. Finally, before taking adaptogens, you'll want to discuss your symptoms with your doctor so you can select the appropriate one for your needs.

Adaptogens need to be timed and dosed correctly throughout the day and adjusted overtime.

FUNCTIONAL ADAPTOGENS

Botanical adaptogens help alleviate stress.

- **Holy Basil (Tulsi):** This adaptogenic herb is helpful to reduce anxiety, lower stress levels, and improve mental clarity. It also shortens the duration of the common cold. You can make or purchase holy basil tea.

- **Ashwagandha:** This evergreen shrub grows in India and comes in powder form. It's helpful for chronic stress and improving working memory and brain function.[15] It also decreases anxiety[16] and systemic inflammation.[17] Some studies show ashwagandha can lower blood sugar levels.[18] It can also increase testosterone levels and fertility in men, making it a natural alternative to Viagra.[19] Ashwagandha can also help your immune system fight off infections and decrease the risk of heart disease by reducing cholesterol and triglyceride levels. Ashwagandha is generally safe, but it's best to check with your health provider if you are taking certain medications.

- **Rhodiola:** This plant grows in Europe and Asia, and its roots are used to improve mood, mental clarity, endurance, and exercise performance. It's suitable for treating stress-induced fatigue. I often recommend rhodiola to patients who complain of exhaustion, sleep issues, or emotional instability.

- **Maca:** This is a popular adaptogen from Peru, great for relieving menopausal symptoms. The supplement comes in powder form, and it's easy to add to a smoothie. It naturally increases estrogen levels, improves stamina, and enhances fertility. In addition, it supports energy and mood. It's also a natural aphrodisiac, particularly for men, supporting overall health and sexual performance.

♦ **Siberian Ginseng:** There are nine different types of ginseng; this information is specific to the Siberian type. It decreases cortisol (stress) production by inhibiting an enzyme known as COMT (catechol-O-methyltransferase). In other words, it keeps your body from having too much cortisol in the bloodstream. So, if you're someone who deals with chronic stress, this can be a helpful adaptogen to take.

♦ **Schisandra Chinensis:** This berry can boost endurance, energy, mental performance and working capacity. In fact, research has found it blocks the formation of excess amyloid plaques, a major component of Alzheimer's disease; therefore, it can be neuroprotective.[20] It also improves liver function and can be helpful in fighting depression. This would be a good supplement for people looking to improve their work performance or optimize their work outs, and/or women going through menopause. You can find it in berry form, as a powder, and as a tea.

Cognitive Support Botanicals

A number of botanicals also support cognitive function by increasing cerebral blood flow and acting as antioxidants and anti-inflammatories. Moreover, these botanicals can positively alter neurotransmitter activity, so if you need improved memory, focus, or clarity, they may be able to help.

COGNITIVE SUPPORT BOTANICALS

- **Bacopa monnieri:** This botanical is suitable for supporting the production of the neurotransmitter GABA. It enhances memory and improves learning and memory acquisition. A study showed that bacopa helped students to retain information better when studying for exams.[21] Bacopa, also known as "herb of grace," is a perennial flower, but it also comes in supplement form.

- **Gotu kola:** This botanical balances the nervous system, improves mental clarity, and accelerates the regeneration of your nerve cells; it also protects the brain from everyday damage, especially neurotoxins like lead, arsenic, and aluminum. It also contains triterpenes that increase the strength and volume of collagen, essential in skin maintenance. You can grow this plant as you would a kitchen herb, in your own yard or pots.

♦ **Rosemary:** Rosemary has a specific effect on blood vessel connective tissue. It enhances circulation by increasing blood supply to the brain. People use rosemary to treat headaches and menstrual pain since it dilates the blood vessels to bring more blood supply to these areas. You'll even see rosemary in shampoos to increase circulation to the scalp and help with hair growth.

♦ **Saffron:** As with rosemary, saffron is often used in foods, has antioxidant and anti-inflammatory properties, and can also be taken as a supplement. It may also inhibit β-amyloid plaque deposition— these are the plaques that deposit in the brain and are the hallmark of Alzheimer's disease. In fact, "numerous studies have found that saffron and turmeric possess the ability to treat patients with Alzheimer's as effectively as conventional treatments."[22] Therapeutic saffron and turmeric are also safer than conventional pharmaceuticals and have less side effects.

♦ **Gingko:** This antioxidant improves the uptake and utilization of oxygen and glucose via the mitochondria in the brain cells. It's often used for people with Alzheimer's and people who have had strokes. Gingko can also reduce anxiety and provide mental flexibility.

♦ **Lion's mane:** Lion's mane is a mushroom you can most likely find at a farmer's market. It stimulates nerve growth factors and reduces oxidative stress. As a result, it's good for mildly improving cognitive function and reducing anxiety and depression.

Nervines, a.k.a. Depression and Anxiety Botanicals

Nervines are botanicals that support your central nervous system and create a sedative effect, making them helpful for people struggling with depression and anxiety. Think of these as the "calm-me-down" botanicals. Particularly for people who deal with high stress, nervines can help restore balance and support restfulness of the body. Nervines act on the CNS limbic system and bind to the GABA receptors, meaning they help calm down your brain activity.

CALMING BOTANICALS, A.K.A. NERVINES

◆ **Lavender:** Lavender's stress-reducing properties are well known. One study says lavender is even comparable to lorazepam, an anti-anxiety drug.[23] It can be taken orally (as a spice, tea, or in capsule form) or breathed in through aromatherapy.

◆ **Kava:** Kava, an evergreen shrub from the Pacific Islands, helps reduce anxiety and can also help usher in sleep. However, if you have liver disease, drink heavily, or are on an antidepressant, approach this one with caution; similar to ibuprofen, kava creates extra work for the liver. Kava is typically ingested via powder form.

◆ **Magnolia bark:** Magnolia bark is an anxiolytic, meaning it "breaks apart anxiety." Besides reducing anxiety, it can be used for headaches, to treat digestive issues, and reduce inflammation. Magnolia can also help improve mood, enhance sleep, and decrease stress. It's usually well tolerated and can be taken in capsule form.

◆ **Lemon balm:** Lemon balm can alleviate symptoms of depression, but it should not be used if you have thyroid issues because it can decrease the production of thyroid hormones. It's typically taken as a tea.

The way you take botanicals will depend on the particular symptoms you want to address; for instance, if you're anxious and struggling to sleep, you may want to take a nervine, whereas if you're anxious and experiencing fatigue while awake, an adaptogen might be better. Once again, I recommend that you talk with a healthcare provider who has expertise in botanicals for recommendations and to understand possible drug interactions.

At the beginning of this chapter, I recommended that you ideally think of supplements as the ornaments that decorate a healthy, green Christmas tree. I encourage you to do everything you can to fuel your body with nutrient-rich foods and apply the recommendations throughout the rest of this book so that you can help yourself grow as that beautiful tree. Once you're ready to add these supplements as your decorations to boost your health, you can take some of the following practical steps.

A RITUAL FOR SUPPLEMENTATION

There's really only one ritual that makes sense for the area of supplements: take them intentionally! People often forget to take their supplements and botanicals because they're not in plain sight. Keeping them organized and visible will help you to remember.

I recommend getting them organized for each day of the week. This is a ritual that I do, personally. I separate my supplements into what I will take with breakfast, lunch, and dinner once a week, so the ritual becomes easy and I remember.

FINDING YOUR BALANCE

Remember: everything in your body's ecosystem works together. Diet, medications, hydration, and supplements all affect your body's ability to absorb nutrients, and it's important to understand how they interact (and their possible side effects). Even your time outside in the sun influences your body's nutritional levels! In addition, many of the hormones, vitamins, and chemicals your body needs can be achieved through some of the other practices discussed in this book. For example, before reaching for one of the anti-anxiety nervine botanicals, you might try going for a hike. Exercise in a natural environment might help your anxiety more than a simple supplement.

The famous integrative medicine pioneer, Dr. Andrew Weil, summed it up when he said, "Millions of Americans today take dietary supplements, practice yoga, and integrate other natural therapies into their lives. These are all preventative measures and can keep people from doctor's offices and reduce the cost of treating serious health issues like heart disease and diabetes." My advice to you as you launch your wellness plan is to concentrate on the preventative measures that will have the most positive impact on your holistic health and happiness. Finally, add a few targeted supplements to your healthy diet and lifestyle.

Reflect on Your #CellCare

Using these guiding questions, take a moment to build self-awareness and reflect on your supplementation needs:

- ♦ Consider what sort of supplements you're taking which do not fall into the category of "whole foods," such as protein powder, vitamins, supplements, and teas. Once you've taken an inventory, consider whether you genuinely need all these forms of supplementation and whether they're helping.

- ♦ Do you think your health would benefit from a consultation with an integrative or functional medicine doctor to identify nutrient deficiencies?

- ♦ Can you address gaps in your nutritional intake through making some minor changes to your food intake, before turning to targeted supplementation?

- ♦ Are there any supplements or botanicals discussed in this chapter that you should research further and look into taking?

THE ANATOMY OF WELLBEING

DESIGN YOUR WELLBEING

In the space below, note your thoughts about how you might want to change your intake of supplements based on what you learned in this chapter.

DESIGN YOUR WELLBEING

Form Your Personalized Four-Week Plan

"The key to forming good habits is to make them part of your 'rituals.' It's one way to bundle good habits into regular times that you set aside to prepare yourself for the life you want."

~ **LEWIS HOWES, AUTHOR OF** THE SCHOOL OF GREATNESS

IF YOU'VE READ THIS FAR, THEN YOU HAVE LEARNED A LOT.

You've learned about how your body and mind work, your nutritional and supplemental needs, the importance of getting movement and sound sleep, the significance of space, processing your emotions, and how to support your body to eliminate toxins.

Now, it's time to translate that knowledge into action. In this final chapter, you'll learn how to design your wellbeing plan for proactive #CellCare. This is the next step in building a sustainable lifestyle that will lead you to greater whole health and wellbeing.

You will be invited to self-reflect and draft your response following every step. You can also find a printable workbook at DrBhanote.com to input your answers in one concise document. Consider printing out your responses and placing them somewhere you'll see them every day to refer to them throughout your wellbeing journey. This plan is totally flexible and is meant to evolve as you go deeper and deeper into your wellbeing. This is not a static "one and done." Be open. Be mindful. And most of all, be intentional. Make this plan work for you as you begin a transformative journey toward greater wellbeing.

YOUR WELLBEING PLEDGE

The first step in taking action begins with a mental decision to try.

My patient, a busy mom of three, was interested in learning how nutrition could support her active, chaotic lifestyle. However, she started by telling me, "Honestly, I just don't have time for self-care. I can't figure out nutritious meals. So I'm just trying to get through the day." At that moment, she had decided that she wasn't going to try.

I suggested, "Why don't you get your kids involved in the process of making food?" That idea hadn't occurred to her—but it was appealing. So she took her kids to the grocery store and enlisted their help picking ingredients. Then, they all worked together that night to prepare a meal. Including her children allowed them to learn some new life skills and also saved her some time. It was a win-win situation, especially when the older daughter and mom discovered a newfound interest in learning to cook and attended my Culinary Medicine Plant-Based Nutrition classes.

Some people believe they're too busy to take action toward wellbeing, but the beauty of rituals is that they can *create* more space and time in your life. For example, this mom was caring for her kids, running errands, and engaging them in activities—but by intentionally working in a ritual of making meals as a family, she's doing all three at once: her kids are being cared for, they're engaged in helping her, and she's still getting her daily task of making dinner completed. By inserting more intentionality throughout her day, she found that her regular tasks took on greater purpose and meaning while helping her family become healthier.

When selecting rituals, I encourage you to develop a plan that works with your lifestyle in an *easy, enjoyable, sustainable* way. But before you can think about how that might work in your own life, it's essential to affirm your decision to try with a pledge to yourself. I invite you to begin your pledge by acknowledging and completing these statements:

MY WELLBEING PLEDGE

I pledge allegiance to the person within and agree to the following:

- I recognize that I could make changes to allow me to live with greater health and happiness.

- I will work on my commitment to my health on most days, or at least five days a week.

- I will spend at least ___ minutes per day on my rituals, or I will complete at least ___ rituals per day.

- If I miss a day, I will _____ ___ in order to make it up.

- I will expect nothing more of myself than to continue making progress.

- I will declare any day I do the above successful, regardless of the result.

- If and when I experience trouble fulfilling the above pledge, I will reread and come back to my intentional practices for my wellbeing.

- Signature and Date:_____

This pledge supports a growth mindset, which we discussed as powerful in Chapter Two. When you recognize that you have the power to change your life and affirm your willingness to try, you've already won half the battle.

YOUR WELLBEING MANIFESTO

To sustain motivation in making these changes, it's crucial to identify an intention behind them. By forming your Wellbeing Manifesto, you'll have the opportunity to connect your lifestyle changes to some of your life's most important decisions. Your Manifesto is a written declaration of what you want in life. It helps you gain clarity and prioritize what is important to you. It can serve as a daily reminder of who you are and what you stand for. Creating a Manifesto can set the foundation for your goals, serve as a source of inspiration every day, and be your compass when you feel lost.

I will share how I have approached lifestyle rituals in my own life. Around fifteen years ago, I felt what many overworked individuals feel: I had too much to do and too little time to do it all. Taking care of patients, taking care of myself, and taking care of my home required daily attention. Trying to do it all was exhausting and sometimes led me to want to let things go. I decided I needed to try to make some changes if I was going to maintain a more sustainable lifestyle as a physician.

Specifically, I wanted to revamp my nutrition. Typically, doctors' lounges provided a small selection of foods to eat during shifts, such as bagels and pastries for breakfast, canned soup and pre-made deli sandwiches for lunch, and whatever is available in the cafeteria for dinner, usually fried foods or pizza. In other words, the menu tended to

THE ANATOMY OF WELLBEING

be nutrient-poor. After years and years of eating hospital food—which I didn't realize had been depleting me of nutrients—I was running on empty. I realized that if I could eat nutrient-dense foods more consistently, then I would likely experience greater overall wellbeing.

So, let's imagine I'm sitting down at home—around fifteen years ago—preparing to write my Wellbeing Manifesto as a way to commit to positive, intentional changes. In writing my Wellbeing Manifesto, I will write down my goals for the future and describe my current state. Then, I'll look at how revamping my food intake will help me achieve my goal. This Manifesto will also prompt me to express my identity so that I'm claiming my power to make these changes in my life: I remember that I am more than just an overworked physician; I am a capable human being, and I am powerful in my ability to make intentional changes.

With all that in mind, here is how I would have written my Wellbeing Manifesto around fifteen years ago when I started this journey.

WELLBEING MANIFESTO: DR. B'S EXAMPLE, CIRCA EARLY 2000S

◆ **My goals for my future** are to help my patients regain health and wellbeing; to create space and time for my self-development, learning, and leisure; and to create a safe, comfortable living environment where I can flourish.

400

- **My purpose is** to bring greater health and wellbeing to everyone in my sphere of influence, prioritizing lifestyle shifts that are sustainable and eco-conscious.

- **My starting point:** Since I eat most of my breakfasts and lunches from the doctors' lounge, I experience energy spikes and lows (which I compensate for with coffee). As a result of these eating habits, I suspect I might be deficient in some nutrients and they are not serving me well.

- **I want to start** finding sustainable ways to improve my nutritional intake that aren't incredibly time-consuming so that I can work more efficiently. For example, it would be great if I could make meal prep fun.

- **The legacy I will leave will be** that I was an amazing physician who consistently improved others' health and wellbeing. I also want to practice what I preach.

- **My identity *does not reside*** behind a desk in a white coat. **The identity I ascribe to myself** is that of a compassionate human being who overcomes the same challenges as my patients with a growth mind-set. Thus, I am able to prioritize my wellbeing and reach my goals, just as I encourage them to do the same.

This was where I started—and it set me in a direction to make slow, steady progress toward greater wellbeing in every area of my life. I was looking at the long game, and as a result, I was able to make consistent changes over time. For example, I went from eating hospital food to ultimately becoming trained in culinary medicine and teaching cooking classes in the community. Eventually, I started a regular yoga practice, became more self-aware of my emotions and peer relationships, and decreased my toxic burden by swapping out products for cleaner alternatives. I also was able to tap more deeply into a growth mindset. I wasn't on autopilot anymore, living life with a conveyor belt of obligations. Instead, I was awake, intentional, and living.

I now track many intentional wellbeing rituals, but I started with just a few. Success in those areas set me on a path to continue building in more and more sustainable rituals. I encourage you to do the same.

In creating a Wellbeing Manifesto, you're mapping out the big picture of how your changes will connect you with the person you want to be. You're identifying your Point A and Point B and naming the purpose behind reaching your Point B. By writing these things down, you build a clear understanding of why your work at making lifestyle changes will be worth the effort. These points will help sustain your motivation and fuel your willingness to take action.

Now it's your turn. Draft some initial answers for your Wellbeing Manifesto. You'll have a chance to hone and revise these throughout your journey.

My Wellbeing Manifesto

♦ My goals for my future

♦ My purpose is

♦ In my current state

♦ I want to start doing _____
   _____ so that I can achieve

♦ I want to leave a legacy of

♦ **My identity *is not***

♦ **My identity *is***

REVIEW YOUR #CELLCARE
REFLECTIONS

Now it's time to decide which area you'd like to change first. Go back through the reflection questions at the end of each chapter in the "Design Your Wellbeing" sections. Was there one significant area you could identify for improvement? Is there any area where you have the most desire to feel healthier and happier?

Next, think about what new practices might help you achieve your goals and become the person you want to be based on the answers you wrote down on your Wellbeing Manifesto. Perhaps you have realized that your nutritional intake is decent, but you're getting almost no physical activity; or maybe you've discovered that your diet could use some serious attention; or you want to focus on getting better sleep because you feel tired all the time. Identify the area of your life that would most benefit from intentional changes and write that down.

If you're still struggling to identify where to start, think about what you'd *enjoy* doing the most. Maybe you've been an athlete for most of your life, but you've gained close to twenty pounds in the past few years. You might enjoy getting back to the physical activity that always felt like such a massive part of you. Or if you love to cook and you know how to get around the kitchen—but you *don't* know how to get around the gym—start in your happy place by cleaning up your nutrition.

Making changes in an area you already associate with positive emotions will make you more likely to maintain those healthy changes. If you can do that, you'll start experiencing a noticeable difference in your health and wellbeing, which will motivate you to take on new rituals and keep the momentum going.

Feel free to write up to two areas you'd like to focus attention on. Try not to name more than two as you begin; otherwise, you may struggle to maintain your plan.

The Area(s) I Choose
to Focus On First

Write down one or two lifestyle areas where you most want to target making changes. This area should be the one that will likely lead to the most noticeable changes in your wellbeing.

SELECT RITUALS TO START WITH

Once you know what one or two areas you'd like to focus on, look through the recommended rituals from the related chapter(s). Then, choose the rituals you'd like to start trying. These should be the ones that feel easiest and most appealing—something that sounds like it would be fun to try.

Easy is essential because it will help transform unintentional habits. Remember, your habits get wired into your brain and your body. To change your habits into ones that will serve you, shift your daily practices ever so slightly in a more intentional direction. For instance, if you're used to drinking coffee every morning, you might consider drinking warm lemon water before your stomach is hit with acidic coffee. In this way, you can build *momentum* along the path of least resistance when you select a ritual that feels easy and doable.

Then, that momentum will usher in a noticeable change; you'll notice that you're starting to feel better and that your new ritual is genuinely serving you. Taking advantage of your positive momentum will allow you to keep moving forward. Your changes, combined with your motivation, will help "rewire" your brain as you build new neural pathways. Suddenly, your daily practices will be powerfully serving you in a way that feels easy.

I'll go back to my example. When I was looking for ways to improve my nutrition, I decided to start taking an evening cooking class at a nearby high school from a vegan nutritionist. I also decided I could simply be more intentional about my food intake. I knew how to cook—I grew up cooking. But despite studying people's cells all day long, I was not intentionally feeding my own body the nutrients it needed to thrive. I decided I could start doing that if I just put in a little thought and effort.

SELECTING RITUAL(S): AN EXAMPLE

My goal is to eat more nutrient-dense foods.

I want to try a cooking class and cook at least one healthy meal a day for myself.

Once you've selected a ritual that you'd like to try, consider where that ritual will fit best into your twenty-four-hour day. Next, make a plan about when you will do your ritual, and remember, if you can layer it onto a pre-existing routine, you may have an easier time keeping it up.

In my example, I had the most available time on the weekends, so that's where I focused the bulk of my meal planning and food prep. I did my grocery shopping on Saturdays and prepared meals on Sundays. I also made myself three days' worth of green juices that I could bring to work with me. My prep and planning enabled me to efficiently make myself healthier dinners on nights when I usually would have only felt capable of pulling something out of the freezer.

If you feel like you don't have *any* available time to try something new, try a different exercise first: write out your typical twenty-four-hour day. Often, we don't even recognize space in our schedules for investing in ourselves because we feel stressed and hurried. But when I ask my patients to write up their typical day, we're almost always able to find a spot for healthy change.

Give this a try for yourself. Draft your ideas about which rituals you might want to try out and where they would best fit your day. Remember to think about the daily rhythms you already have in your life—the customary practices that characterize your twenty-four-hour day. Use these rhythms to help yourself layer in intentional rituals.

RITUAL PLANNING

My goal is

A ritual I want to try is

Here's how I could fit that ritual (or those rituals) into my twenty-four-hour day:

♦ Morning:

♦ Afternoon:

♦ Evening:

♦ Weekends:

Track Your Wellbeing Rituals

Now we're going to get concrete and track your Wellbeing Rituals. You can write these rituals down in this book, in your notebook, or using the printable workbook at DrBhanote.com. Adapt it to work for you and what you're trying to do. Remember: it's important to start with the easiest option. There's no point in going all out, doing *all* the rituals at the same time, if you can't sustain them. Start slow, start intentionally, and focus on building consistency.

> **#CellCare:** Health is not about perfection, but about being intentional and consistent.

Track your Wellbeing Rituals for one month, noting each day of the week. If you want to try several rituals, you might want to break each day into several spots for morning, afternoon, and evening. Next to the time slot where you intend to do the ritual, write the ritual down and why you want to do it. Circle the days when you complete the ritual.

Here is an example of how I tracked my Wellbeing Rituals early in my journey. I only started off with a few, focusing on building consistent progress. Once I was successful in maintaining these, I added in more. Now, I'm up to practicing around twenty rituals a day, but they all feel easy to maintain because they've become part of the enjoyable rhythms of my life.

You will be able to serve your body by, likewise, making one small, sustainable change after another. Remember, slow and steady is key. On Week 1, you may decide you only want to focus on *one* new ritual—perhaps going for an evening walk twice in the first week. Although this might seem so easy as to be insignificant, building momentum with the first ritual is the most important. After successfully completing this first ritual for a week, you will have

My Wellbeing Rituals

MONTH OF : January

MORNING RITUAL

Five minutes of diaphragmatic breathing to start my day on a positive and purposeful note.

	1	2	3	4	5	6	7
8	9	10	11	12	13	14	15
16	17	18	19	20	21	22	23
24	25	26	27	28	29	30	31

AFTERNOON RITUAL

To fuel my cells with the oxygen and movement they require, a gratitude walk of 10,000 steps is the best way for me to recharge my batteries.

	1	2	3	4	5	6	7
8	9	10	11	12	13	14	15
16	17	18	19	20	21	22	23
24	25	26	27	28	29	30	31

EVENING RITUAL

Taking 5 minutes to journal helps me reflect on my day, process my emotions, and visualize the future.

	1	2	3	4	5	6	7
8	9	10	11	12	13	14	15
16	17	18	19	20	21	22	23
24	25	26	27	28	29	30	31

strengthened your motivation (and your neural synapses!) for Week 2. Choose the ritual that sounds like the most fun, the easiest, and the most directly aligned with your target goal for wellbeing. Consider sharing what you're doing with a friend, or even recruiting someone to practice a ritual along with you—this accountability will help your consistency and most likely make your wellbeing journey more fun.

During Week 2, you might add two additional walks, these ones in the morning. These walks might be power walks to get your heart rate up, but maybe you keep them short so that you're maintaining consistency—only a mile. Again, look for rhythms that are already present in your life that you can build on. For example, if you have a daily habit of reading an inspirational book on the couch, listen to the audio version on your headphones instead while incorporating a walk. Keep this process going, slowly adding new rituals once you've been able to consistently practice your first ones.

After four weeks, you will sense a noticeable difference in your energy, focus, and strength. At that point, consider what new rituals you may want to track for the next four weeks, now incorporating new ideas you're excited to try.

This rituals tracker is meant to help you plan for your rituals, hold you accountable for doing them, and affirm and celebrate the successful completion of them. This will help you build powerful momentum for whole health and wellbeing.

Now it's your turn! Create the first draft here, and then check out the digital version available on my website to update or adapt this worksheet as you see fit so that it's as convenient and workable as possible.

My Wellbeing Rituals

MONTH OF : ....

MORNING RITUAL

	1	2	3	4	5	6	7
	8	9	10	11	12	13	14	15
	16	17	18	19	20	21	22	23
	24	25	26	27	28	29	30	31

AFTERNOON RITUAL

	1	2	3	4	5	6	7
	8	9	10	11	12	13	14	15
	16	17	18	19	20	21	22	23
	24	25	26	27	28	29	30	31

EVENING RITUAL

	1	2	3	4	5	6	7
	8	9	10	11	12	13	14	15
	16	17	18	19	20	21	22	23
	24	25	26	27	28	29	30	31

Regardless of how you set up your own process of tracking your Wellbeing Rituals, I encourage you to have some sort of spot that allows you to check the ritual off when you try it out. Sometimes, my patients tell me they failed at one of their rituals. So I'll ask them, "How many times did you try to do it?"

The answer is usually: "Once."

You can't say you failed at something when you gave up after one attempt! That's not trying. Checking off even your attempts at a ritual is important because it creates accountability for your actions.

Remember: you are pursuing behavioral change, which requires your initiative and the responsibility to follow through. Behavioral change is not easy. I've tried to help you find the path of least resistance, but your effort still plays a key role. We began this chapter with your Wellbeing Pledge: it's a commitment to try and try again.

> #**CellCare:** Here's your goal: in whatever area you're working on, do it *one percent* better the next day.

Give it an honest effort. Do your best. You don't have to be perfect—there is no such thing. Your goal should simply be to do better the next day. There's no right or wrong way with this. You're on your unique journey to wellbeing, and ultimately, you're going to discover which path will bring you health and happiness.

413

INSPIRED TO
LEARN MORE?

"The day you plant the seed is not the day you eat the fruit. Be patient and stay the course."

~ FABIENNE FREDRICKSON, AUTHOR

HERE'S MY ENCOURAGEMENT TO YOU: *THE POWER OF RITUALS WORKS.* I have seen this in my own life and the lives of many of my patients. Having tracked my Wellbeing Rituals, I've gathered information that clearly shows how well they work on the days I do them, versus the days I don't. So it's no surprise that when I omit doing a ritual, I feel less than optimal than on the days when I follow it. Mostly though, thanks to the intentional practices I have integrated into my daily rhythms, I practice #CellCare and maximize wellbeing.

> **#CellCare:** A ritual can simplify our everyday lives and enable us to overcome obstacles.

COURSE CORRECT

This book provides you with a compass that I hope has inspired you to become more aware of what you want out of life. Using this Fulfillment Compass, you can navigate your way to wellness by following your motivations and inspirations. When you are willing to step out of your comfort zone, and know that you will alway find your way, it will guide you to success. This compass symbolizes your mindful connection with yourself and the greater universe. As a result, it continuously provides you with direct, real-time information regarding how you feel and what is best for you. When you use this compass to discover your authentic self, you align your beliefs and revitalize your health.

Use the knowledge that you have gained on these pages:

♦ **Power of rituals:** With rituals, you can leverage your brain's neuroplasticity and perform intentional practices to transform your brain and body. I believe this more strongly than ever after using rituals in my healing journey.

FULFILLMENT COMPASS

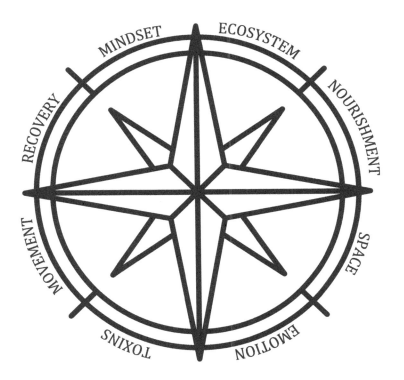

♦ **Transforming your mindset:** Embrace a growth mindset, remembering that your thoughts can be governed and, therefore, your stress response can be managed. Utilize the parasympathetic protocol to train your mind as you become familiar with the brain's stress response.

◆ **Your body's ecosystem:** Your cells, which form the foundation of your entire body, can be fed and nourished intentionally. Keep in mind that everything in the body is connected. By caring for your cellular health and the health of your essential organs, you are setting up your body's ecosystem for wellbeing, both in the short and long-term.

◆ **Culinary nourishment:** You have learned that food can truly be medicine. Use the information you've gained about culinary nourishment to maintain a healthy body.

◆ **Art of movement:** Maintain your fascia, the body's armor, with flexibility exercises; increase your heart health and nutrient flow with aerobic exercise; strengthen your body to increase metabolism; engage your core to make your body more agile and balanced. Moving your body regularly is one of the best ways to make it work harmoniously.

◆ **Restorative recovery:** To ensure that you get a good night's sleep, adopt good sleep hygiene and eliminate sleep saboteurs. Sleep well so that your body can heal and your mind can function at its best.

◆ **Eliminating hidden toxins:** You've learned about some of the main toxic culprits and their sources, and their damaging impact on the body. By taking steps to eliminate some of these toxins, your body's natural toxin-removal systems will perform better, allowing you to operate with a healthier ecosystem.

◆ **Space as sanctuary:** Take ownership of your space. Design a living and working sanctuary utilizing the tools of light, chromotherapy, organization, and scent conducive to optimal wellbeing.

◆ **Emotional exploration:** By building self-awareness and understanding your emotions and "happy hormones," you can foster greater emotional intelligence, which will positively influence your health, spiritual connection, and relationships—all of which have a direct impact on your wellbeing.

◆ **Leveling up:** You've learned to approach supplements with some healthy skepticism and have tools to seek out the supplements that will best serve the nutritional deficiencies in your body. You can enhance physical and mental functions through targeted supplementation that increases performance levels.

The power to restore your cellular health and course-correct toward revitalization lies within you. You can track your daily rhythms—your sleep quality, mood, energy, and so on. Then, by understanding and seeing your body's data, you will be able to connect the dots and make changes that will improve your wellbeing. This power belongs to you. #CellCare is the ultimate biohack!

EMBRACE YOUR UNIQUE JOURNEY

I've sought to provide you with a greater understanding of how your body functions—to appreciate the unique, intricate anatomical processes that are hard at work every second of your life. As you may now realize, your cellular makeup and structure are unique to you and cannot be compared to any other person's. In building this self-awareness, you've become empowered to help protect and nourish your body's ecosystem. Using the tools in this book, you can identify what is best for you and integrate intentional practices each day that will bring health, happiness, and cellular longevity. #CellCare is not a luxury—it's a necessity!

Remember, the wellness industry is worth $4.5 trillion, and there is no shortage of "experts" trying to sell you sunshine. You now have the foundation to move forward with evidence-informed knowledge and understand your body's own inner workings. I hope you feel more empowered to discern what will truly serve your #CellCare.

The pursuit of wellbeing does not come without effort. People rarely discuss the personal investment required for success. A person's image of wellbeing is only the tip of the iceberg—what's outwardly visible is supported by tremendous work that often goes unseen, beneath the surface. The path to wellbeing can be filled with sacrifice, failure, and disappointment. However, there will also be times of courage, persistence, and growth.

Remember, your journey—is *your* journey, and that should be your intention when you embark on it.

As long as you are alive and conscious, you have the power to transform your life. You and I both know there's always something we can do to be a little bit better, and you can start at any time. So take action today and make your wellbeing one percent better than yesterday. Then think how much happier and healthier you will be in a year from now. You are capable of growing, healing, and thriving in unlimited ways. *These are the new rules of wellbeing.*

THE ICEBERG ILLUSION

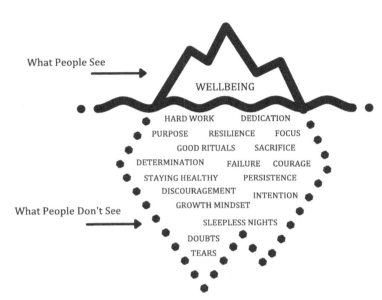

What People See →

WELLBEING

HARD WORK   DEDICATION
PURPOSE   RESILIENCE   FOCUS
GOOD RITUALS   SACRIFICE
DETERMINATION   FAILURE   COURAGE
STAYING HEALTHY   PERSISTENCE
DISCOURAGEMENT   INTENTION
GROWTH MINDSET

What People Don't See →

SLEEPLESS NIGHTS
DOUBTS
TEARS

However—that doesn't mean you have to go on this journey alone.

JOIN WELLKULÅ

Kula, the Sanskrit word for community, brings together individuals who share the same sense of purpose and live with intention. It's an exciting and incredibly powerful thing to pursue wellbeing alongside others. There's commiseration when it's hard, joy when it's fun, and accountability to stick with it. Furthermore, you are more likely to sustain your wellbeing if you are part of a community of others doing it with you.

That's why I want to invite you to join WELLKULÅ: an online community of natural biohackers and practitioners who can help support you on your journey to greater wellbeing. There are several ways to connect:

- ◆ Visit www.DrBhanote.com and subscribe to my news-letter for the latest resources, guides, and events.

- ◆ We invite you to dive deeper into The Anatomy of Well-being (TAOW) through our online training, available at www.DrBhanote.com.

- ◆ Get access to a free mini-course to jumpstart your well-being by sending a copy of your purchase receipt of this book to TAOW@drbhanote.com.

- ◆ Join the global community of natural biohackers inside WELLKULÅ by requesting access to our Facebook group, WELLKULÅ - Lifestyle Design Lab.

- ◆ Connect with me on social media: @drbhanote.

- ◆ I would love to celebrate your progress and be a part of your journey if you tag me: @drbhanote.

- ◆ You can also find like-minded individuals seeking greater wellbeing by using the hashtags #CellCare and #theanatomyofwellbeing.

♦ Have an organization that would benefit from hearing me speak about wellbeing? Email my team at mediainquiries@drbhanote.com.

Remember: *your wellbeing is non-negotiable.* You deserve to flourish, and you are powerful in your ability to infuse your life with intentional practices that serve you. You have what you need to begin your journey toward greater wellbeing. I'll be cheering you on as you embrace your body's unique design and revitalize your health!

LET YOUR CELLS

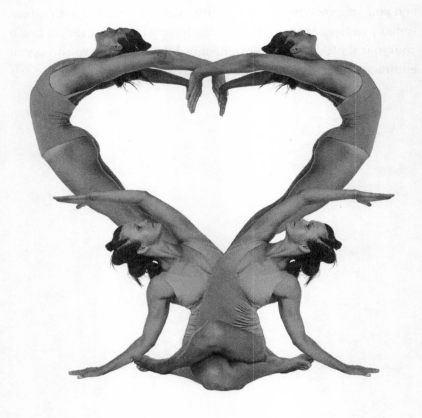

BE YOUR GUIDE

ENDNOTES

INTRODUCTION

1 "Adult Obesity Facts," Centers for Disease Control and Prevention, updated May 17, 2022.

2 "The Health of Millennials," Blue Cross Blue Shield, April 24, 2019.

3 "Wellness Industry Statistics & Facts," Global Wellness Institute, accessed March 30, 2021.

CHAPTER ONE

1 Charles Duhigg, *The Power of Habit: Why We Do What We Do in Life and Business* (St. Louis, MO: Turtleback Books, 2014).

2 Edward L. Bennett et al., "Chemical and Anatomical Plasticity of Brain: Changes in the Brain Through Experience, Demanded by Learning Theories, Are Found in Experiments with Rats," Science 146, no. 3644 (Oct. 30, 1964): 610–619.

3 James Clear, *Atomic Habits: An Easy & Proven Way to Build Good Habits & Break Bad Ones* (New York, NY: Avery, 2018).

4 Clear, *Atomic Habits*.

CHAPTER TWO

1 Sonja Lyubomirsky, Laura King, and Ed Diener, "The Benefits of Frequent Positive Affect: Does Happiness Lead to Success?" *Psychological Bulletin* 131, no. 6 (Nov. 2005): 803–855.

2 Suzanne C. Segerstrom and Gregory E. Miller, "Psychological Stress and the Human Immune System: A Meta-Analytic Study of 30 Years of Inquiry," *Psychological Bulletin* 130, no. 4 (July 2004): 601–630.

3 Claire Eagleson et al., "The Power of Positive Thinking: Pathological Worry Is Reduced by Thought Replacement in Generalized Anxiety Disorder," *Behaviour Research and Therapy* 78 (March 2016): 13–18.

4 Natalie L. Marchant et al., for PREVENT-AD Research Group, "Repetitive Negative Thinking Is Associated with Amyloid, Tau, and Cognitive Decline," *Alzheimer's & Dementia* 16, no. 7 (July 7, 2020): 1054–1064.

5 Hillary Tindle et al., "Optimism, Cynical Hostility, and Incident Coronary Heart Disease and Mortality in the Women's Health Initiative," *Circulation* 120, no. 8 (August 10, 2009): 656–662.

6 Rui Nouchi et al., "Brain Training Game Boosts Executive Functions, Working Memory and Processing Speed in the Young Adults: A Randomized Controlled Trial," *PLoS One* 8, no. 2 (Feb. 6, 2013): e55518.

7 Eileen Luders et al., "Positive Correlations Between Corpus Callosum Thickness and Intelligence," Neuroimage 37, no. 4 (Oct. 1, 2007): 1457–1464.

8 Madhav Goyal et al., "Meditation Programs for Psychological Stress and Wellbeing: A Systematic Review and Meta-Analysis," *JAMA Intern Med.* 174, no, 3 (March 2014): 357–368.

9 Matthew Killingsworth and Daniel T. Gilbert, "A Wandering Mind Is an Unhappy Mind," *Science* 330, no. 6006 (Nov. 12, 2010): 932.

10 Joshua M. Smyth et al., "Online Positive Affect Journaling in the Improvement of Mental Distress and Wellbeing in General Medical Patients with Elevated Anxiety Symptoms: A Preliminary Randomized Controlled Trial," *JMIR Mental Health* 5, no. 4 (Oct.–Dec. 2018): e11290.

11 Bethany E. Kok et al., "How Positive Emotions Build Physical Health: Perceived Positive Social Connections Account for the Upward Spiral Between Positive Emotions and Vagal Tone," *Psychological Science* 24, no. 7 (July 1, 2013): 1123–1132.

CHAPTER THREE

1 Christine Buttorf, Teague Ruder, and Melissa Bauman, "Multiple Chronic Conditions in the United States," Rand Corporation, 2017.

2 Jonathan Lopez and Steven W. G. Tait, "Mitochondrial Apoptosis: Killing Cancer Using the Enemy Within," *British Journal of Cancer* 112, (2015): 957–962.

3 Kashi Raj Bhattarai et al., "Endoplasmic Reticulum (ER) Stress Response Failure in Diseases," *Trends in Cell Biology* 9 (June 16, 2020): 672–675.

4 Denham Harman, "Aging: A Theory Based on Free Radical and Radiation Chemistry," *Journal of Gerontology* 11, no. 3 (July 1956): 298–300.

5 Joseph A. Knight, "Diseases Related to Oxygen-Derived Free Radicals," Annals of Clinical and Laboratory *Science* 25, no. 2 (March–April 1995): 111–121.

6 Lien Ai Pham-Huy, Hua He, and Chuong Pham-Huy, "Free Radicals, Antioxidants in Disease and Health," *International Journal of Biomedical Science* 4, no. 2 (June 2008): 89–96.

CHAPTER FOUR

1 Lori A. Cooper et al., "The Association of Obesity with Sex Hormone–Binding Globulin Is Stronger Than the Association with Ageing – Implications for the Interpretation of Total Testosterone Measurements," *Clinical Endocrinology* 83, no. 6 (Dec. 2015): 828–833.

2 Pedro Carrera-Bastos et al., "The Western Diet and Lifestyle and Diseases of Civilization," *Research Reports in Clinical Cardiology* 2, no. 2 (March 2011): 2–15.

3 Susan M. Krebs-Smith et al., "Americans Do Not Meet Federal Dietary Recommendations," *The Journal of Nutrition* 140, no. 10 (Oct. 2010): 1832–1838.

4 Jessica A. Clark and Craig M. Coopersmith, "Intestinal Crosstalk: A New Paradigm for Understanding the Gut As the 'Motor' of Critical Illness," *Shock* 28, no. 4 (Oct. 2007): 384–393.

5 Yu-Jie Zhang et al., "Impacts of Gut Bacteria on Human Health and Diseases," *International Journal of Molecular Sciences* 16, no. 4 (April 2015): 7493–7519.

6 Pamela Vernocchi, Federica Del Chierico, and Lorenza Putignani, "Gut Microbiota Metabolism and Interaction with Food Components," *International Journal of Molecular Sciences* 21, no. 10 (May 23, 2020): 3688.

7   Amy M. Sheflin et al., "Linking Dietary Patterns with Gut Microbial Composition and Function," *Gut Microbes* 8, no. 2 (2017): 113–129.

8   Yuliya Borre et al., "The Impact of Microbiota on Brain and Behavior: Mechanisms & Therapeutic Potential," *Advances in Experimental Medicine and Biology* 817 (2014): 373–403.

9   Mark Lyte, "Microbial Endocrinology in the Microbiome-Gut-Brain Axis: How Bacterial Production and Utilization of Neurochemicals Influence Behavior," *PLoS Pathogens* 9, no. 11 (Nov. 9, 2013): e1003726.

10   Manuel A. Hernández et al., "The Short-Chain Fatty Acid Acetate in Body Weight Control and Insulin Sensitivity," *Nutrients* 11, no. 8 (Aug. 18, 2019): 1943.

11   Margaret Vourakis, Gaétan Mayer, and Guy Rousseau, "The Role of Gut Microbiota on Cholesterol Metabolism in Atherosclerosis," *International Journal of Molecular Sciences* 22, no. 15 (July 28, 2021): 8074.

12   Dipeeka K. Mandaliya and Sriram Seshadri, "Short Chain Fatty Acids, Pancreatic Dysfunction and Type 2 Diabetes," *Pancreatology* 19, no. 4 (June 2019): 617–622.

13   Hu Liu et al., "Butyrate: A Double-Edged Sword for Health?" *Advances in Nutrition* 9, no. 1 (Jan. 2018): 21–29.

14   T. Sun et al., "Antioxidant Activities of Different Colored Sweet Bell Peppers (Capsicum annuum L.)," *Journal of Food Science* 72, no. 2 (March 12, 2007): S98–102.

15   T. Sun et al., "Antioxidant Activities."

16   Everaldo Attard and Maria-Grazia Martinoli, "Cucurbitacin E, An Experimental Lead Triterpenoid with Anticancer, Immunomodulatory and Novel Effects Against Degenerative Diseases. A Mini-Review," *Current Topics in Medicinal Chemistry* 15, no. 17 (2015): 1708–1713.

17   Wim A. Nijhoff et al., "Effects of Consumption of Brussels Sprouts on Intestinal and Lymphocytic Glutathione S-Transferases in Humans," *Carcinogenesis* 16, no. 9 (Sept. 1995): 2125–2128.

18   Jay H. Fowke, Christopher Longcope, and James R. Hebert, "Brassica Vegetable Consumption Shifts Estrogen Metabolism in Healthy Postmenopausal Women," *Cancer Epidemiology, Biomarkers & Prevention* 9, no. 8 (Aug. 2000): 773–779.

19   Randi L. Edwards et al., "Quercetin Reduces Blood Pressure in Hypertensive Subjects," *The Journal of Nutrition* 137, no. 11 (Nov. 2007): 2405–2411.

20   Genovena Murillo and Rajendra G. Mehta, "Cruciferous Vegetables and Cancer Prevention," *Nutrition and Cancer* 41, no. 1-2 (2001): 17–28.

21   Michael Wien et al., "A Randomized 3×3 Crossover Study to Evaluate the Effect of Hass Avocado Intake on Post-Ingestive Satiety, Glucose and Insulin Levels, and Subsequent Energy Intake in Overweight Adults," *Nutrition Journal* 12, no. 155 (Nov. 27, 2013): 2–9.

22   Terry A. Jacobson, Michael Miller, and Ernst J. Schaefer, "Hypertriglyceridemia and Cardiovascular Risk Reduction," *Clinical Therapeutics* 29, no. 5 (May 2007): 763–777.

23   Shereen N. Mahmood and Whitney P. Bowe, "Diet and Acne Update: Carbohydrates Emerge As the Main Culprit," *Journal of Drugs in Dermatology* 13, no. 4 (April 2014): 428–435.

24   James E. Gangwisch et al., "High Glycemic Index Diet As a Risk Factor for Depression: Analyses from the Women's Health Initiative," *The American Journal of Clinical Nutrition* 102, no. 2 (August 2015): 454–463.

25   Scott E. Kanoski and Terry L. Davidson, "Western Diet Consumption and Cognitive Impairment: Links to Hippocampal Dysfunction and Obesity," *Physiology & Behavior* 103, no. 1 (April 18, 2011): 59–68.

26   Carina C. Montalvany-Antonucci et al., "High-Refined Carbohydrate Diet Promotes Detrimental Effects on Alveolar Bone and Femur Microarchitecture," *Archives of Oral Biology* 86 (Feb. 2018): 101–107.

27   Yujie Xu et al., "Whole grain diet reduces systemic inflammation: A meta-analysis of 9 randomized trials." *Medicine* 97, no. 43 (Baltimore: 2018): e12995.

28   Gang Tang et al., "Meta-Analysis of the Association Between Whole Grain Intake and Coronary Heart Disease Risk," *The American Journal of Cardiology* 115, no. 5 (March 1, 2015): 625–629.

29   Xiao Ma et al., "Association between Whole Grain Intake and All-Cause Mortality: A Meta-Analysis of Cohort Studies," *Oncotarget* 7, no. 38 (September 20, 2016): 61996–62005.

30   Marta Guasch-Ferré et al., "PREDIMED Study Investigators, Dietary Fat Intake and Risk of Cardiovascular Disease and All-Cause Mortality in a Population at High Risk of Cardiovascular Disease," *The American Journal of Clinical Nutrition* 102, no. 6 (December 2015): 1563–1573.

31   Ioannis Delimaris, "Adverse Effects Associated with Protein Intake above the Recommended Dietary Allowance for Adults," *ISRN Nutrition* 2013 (July 18, 2013): 126929.

32   Swapna Upadhyay and Madhulika Dixit, "Role of Polyphenols and Other Phytochemicals on Molecular Signaling," *Oxidative Medicine and Cellular Longevity* 2015 (Dec. 2015): 504253.

33   Anne Rutjes et al., "Vitamin and Mineral Supplementation for Maintaining Cognitive Function in Cognitively Healthy People in Mid and Late Life," *Cochrane Database of Systematic Reviews* 12 (2018): CD011906.

34   Wilhelm Stahl and Helmut Sies, "ß-Carotene and Other Carotenoids in Protection from Sunlight," *The American Journal of Clinical Nutrition* 96, no. 5 (November 2012): 1179S–1184S.

35   Juan Wu et al., "Intakes of Lutein, Zeaxanthin, and Other Carotenoids and Age-Related Macular Degeneration During 2 Decades of Prospective Follow-up," *JAMA Ophthalmology* 133, no. 12 (Dec. 2015): 1415–1424.

36   Keith Griffiths et al., "Food Antioxidants and Their Anti-Inflammatory Properties: A Potential Role in Cardiovascular Diseases and Cancer Prevention," *Diseases* 4, no. 3 (August 2016): 28.

37   Lars Müller et al., "Lycopene and Its Antioxidant Role in the Prevention of Cardiovascular Diseases: A Critical Review," *Critical Reviews in Food Science and Nutrition* 56, no. 11 (August 17, 2016): 1868–1879.

38   Paul F. Jacques et al., "Relationship of Lycopene Intake and Consumption of Tomato Products to Incident CVD," *British Journal of Nutrition* 110, no. 3 (August 28, 2013): 545–551.

39   Joan E. Roberts and Jessica Dennison, "The Photobiology of Lutein and Zeaxanthin in the Eye," *The Journal of Ophthalmology* 2015 (2015): 687173.

40   Richard L. Roberts, Justin Green, and Brandon Lewis, "Lutein and Zeaxanthin in Eye and Skin Health," *Clinics in Dermatology* 27, no. 2 (March–April 2009): 195–201.

41   Michaël G. L. et al., "Flavonoid Intake and Long-Term Risk of Coronary Heart Disease and Cancer in the Seven Countries Study," *Archives of Internal Medicine* 155, no. 4 (February 27, 1995): 381–386. Erratum in: *Archives of Internal Medicine* 155, no. 11 (June 12, 1995): 1184.

42   Pei-Shan Wu et al., "Luteolin and Apigenin Attenuate 4-Hydroxy-2-Nonenal-Mediated Cell Death through Modulation of UPR, Nrf2-ARE and MAPK Pathways in PC12 Cells," *PLoS One* 10, no. 6 (June 18, 2015): e0130599.

43   Ilja C. W. Arts et al., "Catechin Intake Might Explain the Inverse Relation Between Tea Consumption and Ischemic Heart Disease: The Zutphen Elderly Study," *American Journal Clinical Nutrition* 74, no. 2 (August 2001): 227–232.

44   Monira Pervin et al., "Function of Green Tea Catechins in the Brain: Epigallocatechin Gallate and Its Metabolites," *International Journal of Molecular Sciences* 20, no. 15 (July 25, 2019): 3630.

45   Giuseppe Derosa, Pamela Maffioli, and Amirhossein Sahebkar, "Ellagic Acid and Its Role in Chronic Diseases," *Advances in Experimental Medicine and Biology* 928 (2016): 473–479.

46   Nimra Javaid et al., "Neuroprotective Effects of Ellagic Acid in Alzheimer's Disease: Focus on Underlying Molecular Mechanisms of Therapeutic Potential," *Current Pharmaceutical Design* 27, no. 34 (2021): 3591–3601.

47   Tram Kim Lam et al., "Cruciferous Vegetable Consumption and Lung Cancer Risk: A Systematic Review," *Cancer Epidemiol Biomarkers Prev.* 18 no. 1 (2009): 184–195.

48   Walter J. Crinnion, "Organic Foods Contain Higher Levels of Certain Nutrients, Lower Levels of Pesticides, and May Provide Health Benefits for the Consumer," *Alternative Medicine Review* 15, no. 1 (April 2010): 4–12.

49   Nora D. Volkow, George F. Koob, and A. Thomas McLellan, "Neurobiologic Advances from the Brain Disease Model of Addiction," *New England Journal of Medicine* 374, no. 4 (January 28, 2016): 363–371.

50   Paul K. Crane et al., "Glucose Levels and Risk of Dementia," *New England Journal of Medicine* 369, no. 19 (November 7, 2013): 1863–1864.

51   Dongyeop Lee et al., "Effects of Nutritional Components on Aging," *Aging Cell* 14, no. 1 (Feb. 2015): 8–16.

52   Mika Kivimäki et al. "Long-term Inflammation Increases Risk of Common Mental Disorder: A Cohort Study," *Molecular Psychiatry* 19, no. 2 (2014): 149–150.

53   Nataša Tasevska et al., "Sugars in Diet and Risk of Cancer in the NIH-AARP Diet and Health Study," *International Journal of Cancer* 130, no. 1 (2012): 159–169.

54 Stephanie Seneff, Glyn Wainwright, and Luca Mascitelli, "Is the Metabolic Syndrome Caused by a High Fructose, and Relatively Low Fat, Low Cholesterol Diet?" *Archives of Medical Science* 7, no. 1 (Feb. 2011), 8–20.

55 P. A. Todd, P. Benfield, and K. L. Goa, "Guar Gum. A Review of Its Pharmacological Properties, and Use As a Dietary Adjunct in Hypercholesterolaemia," *Drugs* 39, no. 6 (June 1990): 917–928.

56 Alip Borthakur et al., "Prolongation of Carrageenan-induced Inflammation in Human Colonic Epithelial Cells by Activation of an NFκB-BCL10 Loop," *Biochimica et Biophysica Acta* 1822, no. 8 (Aug. 2012): 1300–1307.

57 Kamal Niaz, Elizabeta Zaplatic, and Jonathan Spoor, "Extensive Use of Monosodium Glutamate: A Threat to Public Health?" *EXCLI Journal* 7 (March 18, 2018): 273–278.

58 Food and Drug Law at Keller and Heckman, "OEHHA Releases Report Assessing Potential Neurobehavioral Effects of Synthetic Food Dyes in Children," *National Law Review* 10, no. 245 (Sept. 1, 2020).

59 Ming Ding et al., "Associations of Dairy Intake with Risk of Mortality in Women and Men: Three Prospective Cohort Studies," *BMJ* 367 (2019): l6204.

60 Ding, "Associations of Dairy Intake."

61 Meng Yang et al., "Dietary Patterns after Prostate Cancer Diagnosis in Relation to Disease-Specific and Total Mortality," *Cancer Prevention Research* 8, no. 6 (June 1 2015): 545–551.

62 Gary E. Fraser, et al., "Dairy, Soy, and Risk of Breast Cancer: Those Confounded Milks," *International Journal of Epidemiology* 49, no. 5 (October 2020): 1526–1537.

63 Susan E. McCann et al., "Usual Consumption of Specific Dairy Foods Is Associated with Breast Cancer in the Roswell Park Cancer Institute Data Bank and BioRepository," *Curriculum Developments in Nutrition* 1, no. 3 (February 16, 2017): e000422.

64 Amy Joy Lanou, Susan E. Berkow, and Neal D. Barnard, "Calcium, Dairy Products, and Bone Health in Children and Young Adults: A Reevaluation of the Evidence," *Pediatrics* 115 (2005): 736–743.

65 Jamie Uribarri et al., "Advanced Glycation End Products in Foods and a Practical Guide to Their Reduction in the Diet," *Journal of American Dietetic Association* 110, no. 6 (2010): 911–16.e12.

66 Katherine Hart, "4.6 Fad diets and Fasting for Weight Loss in Obesity," in *Advanced Nutrition and Dietetics in Obesity*, ed. Catherine Hankey (Wiley, 2018), 177–182.

67 Lee Crosby et al., "Ketogenic Diets and Chronic Disease: Weighing the Benefits Against the Risks," *Frontiers in Nutrition* 7 (July 16, 2021): 702802.

68 Akihiko Kitamura et al., "Role Played by Afferent Signals from Olfactory, Gustatory and Gastrointestinal Sensors in Regulation of Autonomic Nerve Activity," *Biological and Pharmaceutical Bulletin* 33, no. 11 (2010): 1778–1782.

69 John D. Teasdale, Zindel Segal, and J. Mark G. Williams. "How Does Cognitive Therapy Prevent Depressive Relapse and Why Should Attentional Control (Mindfulness) Training Help?" *Behaviour Research and Therapy* 33, no. 1 (1995): 25–39.

70 Mehrdad Alirezaei et al., "Short-term Fasting Induces Profound Neuronal Autophagy," *Autophagy* 6, no. 6 (Aug. 6, 2010): 702–710.

71 Bronwen Martin, Mark P. Mattson, and Stuart Maudsleya, "Caloric Restriction and Intermittent Fasting: Two Potential Diets for Successful Brain Aging," *Ageing Research Reviews* 5, no. 3 (Aug. 2006): 332–353.

72 Mark P. Mattson and Ruiqian Wan, "Beneficial Effects of Intermittent Fasting and Caloric Restriction on the Cardiovascular and Cerebrovascular Systems," *The Journal of Nutritional Biochemistry* 16, no. 3 (2005): 129–137.

73 Ken K. Y. Ho et al., "Fasting Enhances Growth Hormone Secretion and Amplifies the Complex Rhythms of Growth Hormone Secretion in Man," *The Journal of Clinical Investigation* 81, no. 4 (April 1988): 968–975.

74 J. Lee et al., "Dietary Restriction Increases the Number of Newly Generated Neural Cells, and Induces Bdnf Expression, in the Dentate Gyrus of Rats," *Journal of Molecular Neuroscience* 15, no. 2 (Oct. 2000): 99–108.

75 T. Aan Jiang, "Health Benefits of Culinary Herbs and Spices," *Journal of AOAC International* 102, no. 2 (March 2019): 395–411.

76 David L. Katz, Kim Doughty, and Ather Ali, "Cocoa and Chocolate in Human Health and Disease," *Antioxidants & Redox Signaling* 15, no. 10 (November 15, 2011): 2779–2811.

77 "Dark Chocolate Consumption Reduces Stress And Inflammation: Data Represent First Human Trials Examining the Impact of Dark Chocolate Consumption on Cognition and Other Brain Functions," Loma Linda University Adventist Health Sciences Center, *ScienceDaily* (April 24, 2018).

78 Eva Martínez-Pinilla, Ainhoa Oñatibia-Astibia, and Rafael Franco, "Relevance of Theobromine for the Beneficial Effects of Cocoa Consumption," *Frontiers in Pharmacology* 6, no. 30 (February 20, 2015).

CHAPTER FIVE

1 Derk-Jan Dijk, "Regulation and Functional Correlates of Slow Wave Sleep," *Journal of Clinical Sleep Medicine* 5, no. 2 (April 15, 2009): S6–15.

2 Susan K. Fried, Dove A. Bunkin, and Andrew S. Greenberg, "Omental and Subcutaneous Adipose Tissues of Obese Subjects Release Interleukin-6: Depot Difference and Regulation by Glucocorticoid," *The Journal of Clinical Endocrinology & Metabolism* 83, no. 3 (March 1998): 847–850.

3 Adam R. Konopka and Matthew P. Harber, "Skeletal Muscle Hypertrophy after Aerobic Exercise Training," *Exercise and Sport Sciences Reviews* 42, no. 2 (2014): 53–61.

4 Frank W. Booth, Christian K. Roberts, and Matthew J. Laye, "Lack of Exercise is a Major Cause of Chronic Diseases," *Comprehensive Physiology* 2, no. 2 (April 2012): 1143–1211.

5 Roald Bahr and Ole M. Sejersted, "Effect of Intensity of Exercise on Excess Postexercise O2 Consumption," *Metabolism.* 40, no. 8 (Aug. 1991): 836–841.

6 Sama F Sleiman et al., "Exercise Promotes the Expression of Brain Derived Neurotrophic Factor (BDNF) Through the Action of the Ketone Body β–hydroxybutyrate," *eLife* 5 (June 2, 2016): e15092.

7 Patrick Z. Liu and Robin Nusslock, "Exercise-Mediated Neurogenesis in the Hippocampus via BDNF," *Frontiers in Neuroscience* 12 (February 7, 2018): 52.

8 Joanna Kruk and Ewa Duchnik, "Oxidative Stress and Skin Diseases: Possible Role of Physical Activity," *Asian Pacific Journal of Cancer Prevention* 15, no. 2 (2014): 561–568.

9 Larry A. Tucker, "Physical Activity and Telomere Length in U.S. Men and Women: An NHANE Investigation," *Preventive Medicine* 100 (2017): 145.

10 C. D. Reimers, G. Knapp, and A. K. Reimers, "Does Physical Activity Increase Life Expectancy? A Review of the Literature," *Journal of Aging Research* 2012 (July 1, 2012): 243958.

11 Scott Powers and Edward T. Howley, *Exercise Physiology: Theory and Application to Fitness and Performance*, 7th ed. (New York: McGraw-Hill Companies, 2009).

12 Brett R. Gordon et al., "The Effects of Resistance Exercise Training on Anxiety: A Meta-Analysis and Meta-Regression Analysis of Randomized Controlled Trials," *Sports Medicine* 47, no. 12 (Dec. 2017): 2521–2532.

13 Ileana Badi, "The Curious Case of Dermal Fibroblasts: Cell Identity Loss May Be a Mechanism Underlying Cardiovascular Aging," *Cardiovascular Research* 115, no. 3 (2019): e24–e25.

14 "Physical Activity Guidelines Resources," *ACSM*, accessed December 9, 2021.

15 Christina Zelano et al., "Nasal Respiration Entrains Human Limbic Oscillations and Modulates Cognitive Function," *Journal of Neuroscience* 36, no. 49 (December 7, 2016): 12448–12467.

16 Xiao Ma et al., "The Effect of Diaphragmatic Breathing on Attention, Negative Affect and Stress in Healthy Adults," *Frontiers in Psychology* 8, no. (June 6, 2017): 874.

17 Catherine Woodyard, "Exploring the Therapeutic Effects of Yoga and its Ability to Increase Quality of Life," *International Journal of Yoga* 4, no. 2 (2011): 49–54.

18 Chris C. Streeter et al., "Effects of Yoga Versus Walking on Mood, Anxiety, and Brain GABA Levels: A Randomized Controlled MRS Study," *Journal of Alternative and Complementary Medicine* 16, no. 11 (2010): 1145–1152.

19 Christopher Kilham, *The Five Tibetans: Five Dynamic Exercises for Health, Energy, and Personal Power* (Rochester, VT: Healing Arts Press, 2011).

20 Miguel García-Jaén et al., "Influence of Abdominal Hollowing Maneuver on the Core Musculature Activation during the Prone Plank Exercise," *International Journal of Environmental Research and Public Health* 17, no. 20 (2020): 7410.

21 Michele Antonelli, Grazia Barbieri, and Davide Donelli, "Effects of Forest Bathing (Shinrin-Yoku) on Levels of Cortisol as a Stress Biomarker: A Systematic Review and Meta-Analysis," *International Journal of Biometeorology* 63, no. 8 (August 2019): 1117–1134.

22 Margaret M. Hansen, Reo Jones, and Kirsten Tocchini, "Shinrin-Yoku (Forest Bathing) and Nature Therapy: A State-of-the-Art Review," *International Journal of Environmental Research and Public Health* 14, no. 8 (July 28, 2017): 851.

23 Peter C. Terry et al., "Effects of Music in Exercise and Sport: A Meta-Analytic Review," *Psychological Bulletin* 146, no. 2 (Feb. 2020): 91–117.

24 Stefan Koelsch et al., "The Impact of Acute Stress on Hormones and Cytokines, and How Their Recovery Is Affected by Music-Evoked Positive Mood," *Scientific Reports* 6, no. 23008 (March 29, 2016).

25 A. Jensen and L. O. Bonde, "The Use of Arts Interventions for Mental Health and Wellbeing in Health Settings," *Perspectives Public Health* 138, no. 4 (July 2018): 209–214.

CHAPTER SIX

1 Natalia Suntsova et al., "Sleep-waking Discharge Patterns of Median Preoptic Nucleus Neurons in Rats," *The Journal of Physiology* 543 (2002): 665–677.

2 Paula Alhola and Päivi Polo-Kantola, "Sleep Deprivation: Impact on Cognitive Performance," *Neuropsychiatric Disease and Treatment* 3 (2007): 553–567.

3 Alhola, "Sleep Deprivation."

4 J. Allan Hobson, "Sleep Is of the Brain, by the Brain and for the Brain," *Nature* 437, no. 7063 (October 27, 2005): 1254–1256.

5 Nancy L. Sin et al., "Sleep Duration and Affective Reactivity to Stressors and Positive Events in Daily Life," *Health Psychology* 39, no. 12 (2020): 1078–1088.

6 Christoph Nissen et al., "Sleep Is More Than Rest for Plasticity in the Human Cortex," *Sleep* 44, no. 33 (March 2021): zsaa216.

7 Nadia Aalling Jessen et al., "The Glymphatic System: A Beginner's Guide," *Neurochemical Research* 40, no. 12 (Dec. 2015): 2583–2599.

8 Andy R. Eugene and Jolanta Masiak, "The Neuroprotective Aspects of Sleep," *MEDtube Science* 3, no. 1 (March 2015): 35–40.

9 Max Hirshkowitz et al., "The National Sleep Foundation's Sleep Time Duration Recommendations: Methodology and Results Summary," *Sleep Health* 1, no. 1 (2015): 40–43.

10 Shalini Paruthi et al., "Recommended Amount of Sleep for Pediatric Populations: A Consensus Statement of the American Academy of Sleep Medicine Academy of Sleep Medicine," *Journal of Clinical Sleep Medicine* 12, no. 6 (2016): 785–786.

11 Nathaniel F. Watson et al., "Recommended Amount of Sleep for a Healthy Adult: A Joint Consensus Statement of the American Academy of Sleep Medicine and Sleep Research Society," *Sleep* 38, no. 6 (2015): 843–844.

12 Amirreza Sajjadieh et al., "The Association of Sleep Duration and Quality with Heart Rate Variability and Blood Pressure," *Tanaffos* 19, no. 2 (2020): 135–143.

13 A. M. Catai et al., "Effects of Aerobic Exercise Training on Heart Rate Variability During Wakefulness and Sleep and Cardiorespiratory Responses of Young and Middle-Aged Healthy Men," *Brazilian Journal of Medical and Biological Research* 35, no. 6 (June 2002): 741–752.

14 Hye-Geum Kim et al., "Stress and Heart Rate Variability: A Meta-Analysis and Review of the Literature," *Psychiatry Investigation* 15, no. 3 (2018): 235–245.

15 Vincent Crasset et al., "Effects of Aging and Cardiac Denervation on Heart Rate Variability During Sleep," *Circulation* 103, no. 1 (January 2, 2001): 84–88.

16 Faye S. Routledge et al., "Improvements in Heart Rate Variability with Exercise Therapy," *Canadian Journal of Cardiology* 26, no. 6 (2010): 303–312.

17 Liye Zou et al., "Effects of Mind-Body Exercises (Tai Chi/Yoga) on Heart Rate Variability Parameters and Perceived Stress: A Systematic Review with Meta-Analysis of Randomized Controlled Trials," *Journal of Clinical Medicine* 7, no. 11 (October 31, 2018): 404.

18 Andrea Zaccaro et al., "How Breath-Control Can Change Your Life: A Systematic Review on Psycho-Physiological Correlates of Slow Breathing," *Frontiers in Human Neuroscience* 12, no. 353 (September 7, 2018).

19 Josie E. Malinowski et al., "The Effects of Dream Rebound: Evidence for Emotion-Processing Theories of Dreaming," *Journal of Sleep Research* 28, no. 5 (Oct. 2019): e12827.

20 Gal Richter-Levin and Irit Akirav, "Amygdala-Hippocampus Dynamic Interaction in Relation to Memory," *Molecular Neurobiology* 22, (2000): 11–20.

21 Liese Exelmans and Jan Van den Bulck, "Bedtime, Shuteye Time and Electronic Media: Sleep Displacement is a Two-Step Process," *Journal of Sleep Research* 26, no. 3 (June 2017): 364–370.

22 Exelmans and den Bulck, "Bedtime."

23 Chloe J. Andre, Victoria Lovallo, and Rebecca M. C. Spencer, "The Effects of Bed Sharing on Sleep: From Partners to Pets," *Sleep Health* 7, no. 3 (June 2021): 314–323.

24 Exelmans and den Bulck, "Bedtime."

25 Catherine E. Milner and Kimberly A. Cote, "Benefits of Napping in Healthy Adults: Impact of Nap Length, Time of Day, Age, and Experience with Napping," *Journal of Sleep Research* 18, no. 2 (June 2009): 272–281.

26 L. G. Aspinwall and S. E. Taylor, "A Stitch in Time: Self-Regulation and Proactive Coping," *Psychological Bulletin* 121, no. 3 (May 1997): 417–436.

27 Shahab Haghayegh et al., "Before-Bedtime Passive Body Heating by Warm Shower or Bath to Improve Sleep: A Systematic Review and Meta-Analysis," *Sleep Medicine Reviews* 46 (August 2019): 124–135.

CHAPTER SEVEN

1 "Opinion on Fragrance Allergens in Cosmetic Products," Scientific Committee on Consumer Safety, European Commission (2012): 33–38.

2 "Not So Sexy: Hidden Chemicals in Perfume and Cologne," Environmental Working Group (2010).

3 P. Kumar, et al., "Inhalation Challenge Effects of Perfume Scent Strips in Patients With Asthma," *Annals of Allergy Asthma Immunology* 75 (1995): 429–433.

4 Lambert Ayuk-Takem et al., "Inhibition of Polyisoprenylated Methylated Protein Methyl Esterase by Synthetic Musks Induces Cell Degeneration," *Environmental Toxicology*, 29, no. 4 (2014): 466–477.

5 "Report on Carcinogens NTP (National Toxicology Program)," 13th ed. U.S. Department of Health and Human Services, Public Health Service (Oct. 2014).

6 David H. Phillips and Volker M. Arlt, "Genotoxicity: Damage to DNA and Its Consequences," EXS 99 (2009): 87–110.

7 Koji Ueda, "Effect of Environmental Chemicals on the Genes and the Gene Expression" trans., Yakugaku Zasshi: *Journal of the Pharmaceutical Society of Japan* 129, no. 12 (Dec. 2009): 1501–1506.

8 Jun Li et al., "Exposure to Polycyclic Aromatic Hydrocarbons and Accelerated DNA Methylation Aging," *Environmental Health Perspectives* 126, no. 6 (June 14, 2018): 067005.

9 Margaret E. Sears, Kathleen J. Kerr, and Riina I. Bray, "Arsenic, Cadmium, Lead, and Mercury in Sweat: A Systematic Review," *Journal of Environmental and Public Health* 2012 (2012): 184745.

10   Dorothy A. Kieffer, Roy J. Martin, and Sean H. Adams, "Impact of Dietary Fibers on Nutrient Management and Detoxification Organs: Gut, Liver, and Kidneys," *Advances in Nutrition* 7, no. 6 (November 15, 2016): 1111–1121.

11   Omayma Ar Abo-Zaid et al., "Bisphenol-A/Radiation Mediated Inflammatory Response Activates EGFR/KRAS/ERK1/2 Signaling Pathway Leads to Lung Carcinogenesis Incidence," *International Journal of Immunopathology and Pharmacology* 36, no. 3946320221092918 (Jan.–Dec., 2022).

12   Tristan Hampe et al., "A Comparative In Vitro Study on Monomer Release from Bisphenol A-Free and Conventional Temporary Crown and Bridge Materials," *European Journal of Oral Sciences* 129, no. 6 (Dec. 2021): e12826.

13   Evanthia Diamanti-Kandarakis et al., "Endocrine-Disrupting Chemicals: An Endocrine Society Statement," *Endrocrine Reviews* 30, no. 4 (June 2009): 293–342; Endrocrine Society, "Endrocrine-Disrupting Chemicals: An Endrocrine Society Position Statement," Endrocrine Society, May 1, 2018; Andrea C. Gore et al., "EDC-2: The Endocrine Society's Second Scientific Statement on Endocrine-Disrupting Chemicals," *Endocrine Reviews* 36, no. 6 (Dec. 2015): E1–E150.

14   Ashley J. Malin et al. "Fluoride Exposure and Sleep Patterns Among Older Adolescents in the United States: A Cross-Sectional Study of NHANES 2015–2016," *Environmental Health* 18, no. 1 (2019): 106.

15   International Academy of Oral Medicine and Technology (IAOMT), *Fluoride Exposure and Human Health Risks: A Fact Sheet from the IAOMT* (IAOMT 2017).

16   Julia Green Brody et al., "Breast Cancer Risk and Historical Exposure to Pesticides from Wide-Area Applications Assessed with Gis," *Environmental Health Perspectives* 112, no. 8 (2004): 889–897.

17   Claudine M. Samanic et al., "Occupational Exposure to Pesticides and Risk of Adult Brain Tumors," *American Journal of Epidemiology* 167, no. 8 (2008): 976–985.

18   Camille Ragin et al., "Farming, Reported Pesticide Use, and Prostate Cancer," *American Journal of Men's Health* 7, no. 2 (2013): 102–109.

19   Dan Luo et al., "Exposure to Organochlorine Pesticides and Non-Hodgkin Lymphoma: A Meta-Analysis of Observational Studies," *Scientific Reports* 6, no. 25768 (May 17, 2016).

20   Note: As a consumer, I was not compensated or given any perk to endorse these brands or products.

21   Hartmut Göbel et al., "Oleum Menthae Piperitae (Pfefferminzöl) in der Akutther-apie des Kopfschmerzes vom Spannungstyp [Peppermint Oil in the Acute Treatment of Tension-Type Headache]," *Schmerz* 30, no. 3 (June 2016): 295–310.

22   B. C. Wolverton, Anne Johnson, and Keith Bounds, "Interior Landscape Plants for Indoor Air Pollution Abatement (Report)," NASA (September 1989).

23   Q. Li et al., "Forest Bathing Enhances Human Natural Killer Activity and Expres-sion of Anti-Cancer Proteins," *International Journal of Immunopathology and Phar-macology* 20, no. 2 (2007): 3–8.

24   Cecilia U. D. Stenfors et al., "Positive Effects of Nature on Cognitive Performance Across Multiple Experiments: Test Order but Not Affect Modulates the Cognitive Ef-fects," *Frontiers in Psychology* 10, no 1413 (July 3, 2019).

25   Negar Jamshidi and Marc M. Cohen, "The Clinical Efficacy and Safety of Tulsi in Humans: A Systematic Review of the Literature," *Evidence-Based Complementary and Alternative Medicine* 2017: 9217567 (2017).

26   Michael Boschmann et al., "Water-induced Thermogenesis," *The Journal of Clin-ical Endocrinology and Metabolism* 88, no. 12 (Dec. 2003): 6015–6019.

27   Zhi-Yong Zhang, Xian-Jin Liu, and Xiao-Yue Hong, "Effects of Home Preparation on Pesticide Residues in Cabbage," Food Control 18, no. 12 (2007): 1484–1487.

28   Tianxi Yang, et al. "Effectiveness of Commercial and Homemade Washing Agents in Removing Pesticide Residues on and in Apples," *Journal of Agricultural and Food Chemistry* 65, no. 44 (2017): 9744–9752.

29   Elmar Wienecke and Claudia Nolden, "Langzeit-HRV-Analyse zeigt Stressreduk-tion durch Magnesiumzufuhr [Long-Term HRV Analysis Shows Stress Reduction by Magnesium Intake]," *MMW Fortschritte der Medizin* 158, suppl. 6 (Dec. 2016): 12–16.

30   Jari A. Laukkanen, Tanjaniina Laukkanen, and Setor K. Kunutsor, "Cardiovas-cular and Other Health Benefits of Sauna Bathing: A Review of the Evidence," *Mayo Clinic Proceedings* 93, no. 8 (2018): 1111.

CHAPTER EIGHT

1   Darby E. Saxbe and Rena Repetti, "No Place Like Home: Home Tours Correlate with Daily Patterns of Mood and Cortisol," *Personality and Social Psychology Bulletin* 36, no. 1 (2010): 71–81.

2   Catherine A. Roster, Joseph R. Ferrari, and M. Peter Jurkat, "The Dark Side of Home: Assessing Possession 'Clutter' on Subjective Wellbeing," *Journal of Environmental Psychology* 46 (June 2016): 32–41.

3   Indiana University, "Tidy House, Fitter Body?" *ScienceDaily*, June 3, 2010.

4   Joseph R. Ferrari, "Delaying Disposing: Examining the Relationship between Procrastination and Clutter across Generations," *Current Psychology* 37 (May 2018): 426–431.

5   Stephanie McMains and Sabine Kastner, "Interactions of Top-Down and Bottom-Up Mechanisms in Human Visual Cortex," *Journal of Neuroscience* 31, no. 2 (January 12, 2011): 587–597.

6   Kathleen D. Vohs, Joseph P. Redden, and Ryan Rahinel, "Physical Order Produces Healthy Choices, Generosity, and Conventionality, Whereas Disorder Produces Creativity," *Psychological Science* 24, no. 9 (2013): 1860–1867.

7   Marie Kondo, *Spark Joy: An Illustrated Master Class on the Art of Organizing and Tidying Up* (New York: Ten Speed Press, 2016).

8   Helen L. Walls, Kelvin L. Walls, and Geza Benke, "Eye Disease Resulting from Increased Use of Fluorescent Lighting as a Climate Change Mitigation Strategy," *American Journal of Public Health* 101, no. 12 (2011).

9   Swami Sadashiva Tirtha, *The Āyurveda Encyclopedia: Natural Secrets to Healing, Prevention & Longevity* (Bayville: Ayurveda Holistic Center Press, 2005).

10   Somia Gul, Rabia Khalid Nadeem, and Amun Aslam, "Chromo Therapy: An Effective Treatment Option or Just a Myth?? Critical Analysis on the Effectiveness of Chromo Therapy," *American Research Journal of Pharmacy* 1, no. 2 (Jan. 2015): 62–70.

11   Mindy Green, *Natural Perfumes: Simple, Sensual, Personal Aromatherapy Recipes* (Interweave Press, 1999).

12   Min-sun Lee et al., "Interaction with Indoor Plants May Reduce Psychological and Physiological Stress by Suppressing Autonomic Nervous System Activity in Young Adults: A Randomized Crossover Study," *Journal of Physiological Anthropology* 34, no. 21 (2015).

13   Yun-Ah Oh, Seon-Ok Kim, and Sin-Ae Park, "Real Foliage Plants as Visual Stimuli to Improve Concentration and Attention in Elementary Students," *International Journal of Environmental Research and Public Health* 16, no, 5 (March 5, 2019): 796.

14 Hyunju Jo, Chorong Song, and Yoshifumi Miyazaki, "Physiological Benefits of Viewing Nature: A Systematic Review of Indoor Experiments," *International Journal of Environmental Research and Public Health* 16, no. 23 (2019): 4739.

15 Marlon Nieuwenhuis et al., "The Relative Benefits of Green Versus Lean Office Space: Three Field Experiments," *Journal of Experimental Psychology: Applied* 20, no. 3 (2014): 199–214.

16 Adam W. Hanley et al., "Washing Dishes to Wash the Dishes: Brief Instruction in an Informal Mindfulness Practice," *Mindfulness* 6, no. 5 (2015): 1095–1103.

17 Elizabeth Varney and Jane Buckle, "Effect of Inhaled Essential Oils on Mental Exhaustion and Moderate Burnout: A Small Pilot Study," *Journal of Alternative and Complementary Medicine* 19, no. 1 (Jan. 2013): 69–71.

18 Benjamin J. Malcolm and Kimberly Tallian, "Essential Oil of Lavender in Anxiety Disorders: Ready for Prime Time?" *Mental Health Clinician* 7, no. 4 (2018): 147–155.

19 Dennis Anheyer et al., "Herbal Medicines for Gastrointestinal Disorders in Children and Adolescents: A Systematic Review," *Pediatrics* 139, no. 6 (June 2017): e20170062.

20 Jie Shao et al., "Effects of Different Doses of Eucalyptus Oil from Eucalyptus globulus Labill on Respiratory Tract Immunity and Immune Function in Healthy Rats," *Frontiers in Pharmacology* 11, no. 12872020 (2020).

21 Rafie Hamidpour et al., "Frankincense (rǔ xiāng (boswellia species): From the Selection of Traditional Applications to the Novel Phytotherapy for the Prevention and Treatment of Serious Diseases," *Journal of Traditional and Complementary Medicine* 3, no. 4 (2013): 221–226.

22 Janice K. Kiecolt-Glaser et al., "Olfactory Influences on Mood and Autonomic, Endocrine, and Immune Function," *Psychoneuroendocrinology* 33, no. 3 (April 2008): 328–339.

23 "Cleaning 'Improves Mental Health,'" BBC News, April 9, 2008.

CHAPTER NINE

1 Bethany E. Kok et al., "How Positive Emotions Build Physical Health: Perceived Positive Social Connections Account for the Upward Spiral Between Positive Emotions and Vagal Tone," *Psychological Science* 24, no. 7 (July 1, 2013): 1123–1132.

2   Randy A. Sansone and Lori A. Sansone, "Sunshine, Serotonin, and Skin: A Partial Explanation for Seasonal Patterns in Psychopathology?" *Innovations in Clinical Neuroscience* 10, nos. 7–8 (2013): 20–24.

3   Ulrica Nilsson, "Soothing Music Can Increase Oxytocin Levels During Bed Rest after Open-Heart Surgery: A Randomised Control Trial," *Journal of Clinical Nursing* 18, no, 15 (Aug. 2009): 2153–2161.

4   N. Jayaram et al., "Effect of Yoga Therapy on Plasma Oxytocin and Facial Emotion Recognition Deficits in Patients of Schizophrenia," *Indian Journal of Psychiatry* 55, Supplement 3 (2013): S409–S413.

5   Melissa G. Hunt et al., "No More FOMO: Limiting Social Media Decreases Loneliness and Depression," *Journal of Social and Clinical Psychology* 37, no. 10 (Nov. 2018): 751–768.

6   Nora D. Volkow et al., "Evaluating Dopamine Reward Pathway in ADHD: Clinical Implications," *JAMA* 302, no. 10 (2009): 1084–1091.

7   Tiina Saanijoki et al., "Opioid Release after High-Intensity Interval Training in Healthy Human Subjects," *Neuropsychopharmacology* 43 (2018): 246–254.

8   Ji-Sheng Han, "Acupuncture and Endorphins," *Neuroscience Letters* 361, nos. 1–3 (May 6, 2004): 258–261.

9   Nigel Mathers, "Compassion and the Science of Kindness: Harvard Davis Lecture 2015," *British Journal of General Practice* 66, no. 648 (2016): e525–e527.

10   Takeo Tsujii, Kazutoshi Komatsu, and Kaoru Sakatani, "Acute Effects of Physical Exercise on Prefrontal Cortex Activity in Older Adults: A Functional Near-Infrared Spectroscopy Study," *Advances in Experimental Medicine and Biology* 765 (2013): 293–298.

11   Robert Plutchik, "The Nature of Emotions: Clinical Implications," in *Emotions and Psychopathology*, eds. Manfred Clynes and Jaak Panksepp (Boston, MA: Springer, 1988).

12   Heather S. L. Jim et al., "Religion, Spirituality, and Physical Health in Cancer Patients: A Meta-Analysis," *Cancer* 121, no. 21 (November 1, 2015): 3760–3768.

13   Mohammadreza Hojat, "Human Connection in Health and Illness," in *Empathy in Patient Care* (New York: Springer, 2007).

14   Dan Buettner, *The Blue Zones: 9 Lessons for Living Longer from the People Who've Lived the Longest* (Washington, D.C.: National Geographic, 2012).

15 Gaétan Chevalier et al., "Earthing: Health Implications of Reconnecting the Human Body to the Earth's Surface Electrons," *Journal of Environmental and Public Health* 2012 (Jan. 12, 2012): 291541.

16 James L. Oschman, "Perspective: Assume a Spherical Cow: The Role of Free or Mobile Electrons in Bodywork, Energetic and Movement Therapies," *Journal of Bodywork and Movement Therapies* 12, no. 1 (Jan. 2008): 40–57.

17 Stefan G. Hofmann, Paul Grossman, and Devon E. Hinton, "Loving-Kindness and Compassion Meditation: Potential for Psychological Interventions," *Clinical Psychology Review* 31, no. 7 (2011): 1126–1132.

18 Theresa Van Lith, "Art Therapy in Mental Health: A Systematic Review of Approaches and Practices," *The Arts in Psychotherapy* 47 (Feb. 2016): 9–22.

19 Megan E. Beerse et al., "Biobehavioral Utility of Mindfulness-Based Art Therapy: Neurobiological Underpinnings and Mental Health Impacts," *Experimental Biology and Medicine* 245, no. 2 (Jan. 2020): 122–130.

20 Girija Kaimal, Kendra Ray, and Juan Muniz, "Reduction of Cortisol Levels and Participants' Responses Following Art Making," *Art Therapy* 33, no. 2 (April 2, 2016): 74–80.

21 Hunt et al., "No More FOMO."

CHAPTER TEN

1 Chung S. Yang, Joshua D. Lambert, and Shengmin Sang, "Antioxidative and Anti-Carcinogenic Activities of Tea Polyphenols," *Archives of Toxicology* 83, no. 1 (2009): 11–21.

2 Qian Yi Eng, Punniyakoti Veeraveedu Thanikachalam, and Srinivasan Ramamurthy, "Molecular Understanding of Epigallocatechin Gallate (Egcg) in Cardiovascular and Metabolic Diseases," *Journal of Ethnopharmacology* 210 (January 10, 2018): 296–310.

3 Keiko Unno et al., "Anti-Stress Effect of Green Tea with Lowered Caffeine on Humans: A Pilot Study," *Biological and Pharmaceutical Bulletin* 40, no. 6 (2017): 902–909.

4 Layal Slika and Digambara Patra, "Traditional Uses, Therapeutic Effects and Recent Advances of Curcumin: A Mini-Review," *Mini-Reviews in Medicinal Chemistry* 20, no. 12 (2020): 1072–1082.

5   Ga-Young Choi et al., "Curcumin Alters Neural Plasticity and Viability of Intact Hippocampal Circuits and Attenuates Behavioral Despair and COX-2 Expression in Chronically Stressed Rats," *Mediators of Inflammation* 2017 (2017): 6280925.

6   Binu Chandran and Ajay Goel, "A Randomized, Pilot Study to Assess the Efficacy and Safety of Curcumin in Patients with Active Rheumatoid Arthritis," *Phytotherapy Research* 26, no. 11 (Nov. 2012): 1719–1725.

7   Glyn Howatson et al., "Effect of Tart Cherry Juice (Prunus Cerasus) on Melatonin Levels and Enhanced Sleep Quality," *European Journal of Nutrition* 51, no. 8 (Dec. 2012): 909–916.

8   Elias E Mazokopakis et al., "The Hypolipidaemic Effects of Spirulina (Arthrospira Platensis) Supplementation in a Cretan Population: A Prospective Study," *Journal of the Science of Food and Agriculture* 94, no. 3 (Feb. 2014): 432–437.

9   Marco A. Juárez-Oropeza et al., "Effects of Dietary Spirulina on Vascular Reactivity," *Journal of Medicinal Food* 12, no. 1 (Feb. 2009): 15–20.

10   Chao-Ming Shih et al., "Antiinflammatory and Antihyperalgesic Activity of C-Phycocyanin," *Anesthesia & Analgesia* 108, no. 4 (April 2009): 1303–1310.

11   Takuya Uchikawa et al., "Enhanced Elimination of Tissue Methylmercury in Parachlorella Beijerinckii-Fed Mice," *Journal of Toxicological Sciences* 36, no. 1 (Jan. 2011): 121–126.

12   Uchikawa et al., "Enhanced Elimination."

13   Na Hee Ryu et al., "Impact of Daily Chlorella Consumption on Serum Lipid and Carotenoid Profiles in Mildly Hypercholesterolemic Adults: A Double-Blinded, Randomized, Placebo-Controlled Study," *Nutrition Journal* 13, no. 57 (June 11, 2014).

14   Alexander Panossian and Georg Wikman, "Effects of Adaptogens on the Central Nervous System and the Molecular Mechanisms Associated with Their Stress—Protective Activity," *Pharmaceuticals* 3, no. 1 (2010): 188–224.

15   Dnyanraj Choudhary, Sauvik Bhattacharyya, and Sekhar Bose, "Efficacy and Safety of Ashwagandha (Withania somnifera (L.) Dunal) Root Extract in Improving Memory and Cognitive Functions," *Journal of Dietary Supplements* 14, no. 6 (November 2, 2017): 599–612.

16   Jessica M. Gannon et al., "Effects of a Standardized Extract of Withania Somnifera (Ashwagandha) on Depression and Anxiety Symptoms in Persons with Schizophrenia Participating in a Randomized, Placebo-Controlled Clinical Trial," *Annals of Clinical Psychiatry* 31, no. 2 (May 2019): 123–129.

17 Emilie Logie and Wim Vanden Berghe, "Tackling Chronic Inflammation with Withanolide Phytochemicals—A Withaferin a Perspective," *Antioxidants* 9, no. 11 (2020): 1107.

18 Sharanbasappa Durg, Sachin Bavage, and Shivakumar B. Shivaram, "Withania Somnifera (Indian Ginseng) in Diabetes Mellitus: A Systematic Review and Meta-Analysis of Scientific Evidence from Experimental Research to Clinical Application," *Phytotherapy Research* 34, no. 5 (May 2020): 1041–1059.

19 Adrian L. Lopresti, Peter D. Drummond, and Stephen J. Smith, "A Randomized, Double-Blind, Placebo-Controlled, Crossover Study Examining the Hormonal and Vitality Effects of Ashwagandha (Withania Somnifera) in Aging, Overweight Males," *American Journal of Men's Health* 13, no. 2 (2019): 1557988319835985.

20 Ming Zhang et al., "The Influence of Schisandrin B on a Model of Alzheimer's Disease Using β-amyloid Protein Aβ1-42-mediated Damage in SH-SY5Y Neuronal Cell Line and Underlying Mechanisms," *Journal of Toxicology and Environmental Health* 80, no. 22 (2017): 1199–1205.

21 Navneet Kumar et al., "Efficacy of Standardized Extract of Bacopa Monnieri (Bacognize®) on Cognitive Functions of Medical Students: A Six-Week, Randomized Placebo-Controlled Trial," *Evidence-Based Complementary and Alternative Medicine* 2016 (Oct. 2016): 4103423.

22 Nur Adalier and Heath Parker, "Vitamin E, Turmeric and Saffron in Treatment of Alzheimer's Disease," *Antioxidants* 5, no. 4 (October 25, 2016): 40.

23 H. Woelk and S. Schläfke, "A Multi-Center, Double-Blind, Randomised Study of the Lavender Oil Preparation Silexan in Comparison to Lorazepam for Generalized Anxiety Disorder," *Phytomedicine* 17, no. 2 (Feb. 2010): 94–99.

ABOUT THE AUTHOR

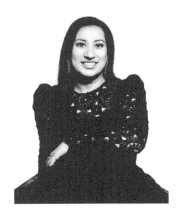

MONISHA BHANOTE, MD, FCAP, ABOIM, IS ONE OF THE FEW quintuple board-certified physicians in the nation. Through her expertise as a cytopathologist, functional culinary medicine specialist, and integrative lifestyle medicine doctor, she combines ancient wisdom with mind-body science to naturally biohack the human body. Dr. Bhanote, known as the Wellbeing Doctor, has diagnosed over one million cancer cases, provides health programs at DrBhanote.com, and leads wellness workshops and retreats worldwide. Featured in *Shape Magazine*, *Reader's Digest,* and *Martha Stewart Living*, Dr. Bhanote serves on several clinical advisory boards and is a go-to health and wellness expert for *Healthline, Psych Central,* and *Medical News Today*. In addition to living on three continents and speaking seven languages, she has traveled to more than fifty countries to explore the latest plant-based recipes and wellness trends.

Made in the USA
Las Vegas, NV
09 December 2024

13670158R10277